'For anyone questioning their relationship with alcohol, this book is a must-read. It's empathetic, inspiring and full of practical ideas and tools that might just change your life.'

Zoe Blaskey, founder of Motherkind

'By exploring the deeper meanings behind why women drink, Sarah Rusbatch helps women find new ways to cope with the complexities of their lives and offers hope, clarity and a new path forward.'

Dr Wendy Sweet PhD, creator of the My Menopause Transformation program

'With a deeply personal and compassionate approach, Sarah leaves no stone unturned when it comes to breaking through the barriers to cutting down on alcohol. She explores the root causes, asks the tough questions, and provides lasting and life-enriching solutions. I recommend Sarah's book to all my patients who want to change their relationship with alcohol and discover their best selves.'

Dr Helena Popovic MBBS, medical practitioner, leading authority on brain health and bestselling author

T0333519

BEYOND BOOZE

How to create a life you love, alcohol-free

SARAH RUSBATCH

murdoch books

Sydney | London

Published in 2024 by Murdoch Books, an imprint of Allen & Unwin

Copyright © Sarah Rusbatch 2024

All rights reserved. No part of this book may be reproduced or transmitted in any form or by any means, electronic or mechanical, including photocopying, recording or by any information storage and retrieval system, without prior permission in writing from the publisher. The Australian *Copyright Act 1968* (the Act) allows a maximum of one chapter or 10 per cent of this book, whichever is the greater, to be photocopied by any educational institution for its educational purposes provided that the educational institution (or body that administers it) has given a remuneration notice to the Copyright Agency (Australia) under the Act.

Murdoch Books Australia
Cammeraygal Country
83 Alexander Street, Crows Nest NSW 2065
Phone: +61 (0)2 8425 0100
murdochbooks.com.au
info@murdochbooks.com.au

Murdoch Books UK
Ormond House, 26–27 Boswell Street, London WC1N 3JZ
Phone: +44 (0) 20 8785 5995
murdochbooks.co.uk
info@murdochbooks.co.uk

 A catalogue record for this book is available from the National Library of Australia

A catalogue record for this book is available from the British Library

ISBN 978 1 76150 008 4

Cover and text design by Christa Moffitt

Typeset by Midland Typesetters, Australia
Printed and bound by CPI Group (UK) Ltd, Croydon CR0 4YY

DISCLAIMER: The content presented in this book is meant for inspiration and informational purposes only. The purchaser of this book understands that the author is not a medical professional, and the information contained within this book is not intended to replace medical advice or to be relied upon to treat, cure or prevent any disease, illness or medical condition. It is understood that you will seek full medical clearance by a licensed physician before making any changes mentioned in this book. The author and publisher claim no responsibility to any person or entity for any liability, loss or damage caused or alleged to be caused directly or indirectly as a result of the use, application or interpretation of the material in this book.

Every reasonable effort has been made to trace the owners of copyright materials in this book, but in some instances this has proven impossible. The author(s) and publisher will be glad to receive information leading to more complete acknowledgements in subsequent printings of the book and in the meantime extend their apologies for any omissions.

We acknowledge that we meet and work on the traditional lands of the Cammeraygal people of the Eora Nation and pay our respects to their elders past, present and future.

10 9 8 7

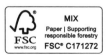 The paper in this book is FSC® certified. FSC® promotes environmentally responsible, socially beneficial and economically viable management of the world's forests.

For all the women reading this book:
I see you,
I honour you,
I am you.

CONTENTS

MY STORY SO FAR ...

'Hobbies?' I scoffed, as I reached over to pour myself another glass of sav blanc. 'And spare time? Don't make me laugh! What woman in her 40s, raising kids, working and running a house has any spare time for hobbies?

'And besides,' I added, 'I have my favourite hobby right here!' I smirked as I made an over-the-top gesture of sniffing my wine, taking a large gulp and letting it swill around my mouth, looking up to the sky and pretending to absorb the flavours of our 'three for $20' bargain.

It was December 2016, a hot Friday afternoon, and I was sitting in my friend Beccy's back garden. I'd been there since school finished, the wine was flowing, the kids were playing, and we were waiting for the pizza to arrive, much the same as any other Friday.

Once again, I'd exceeded my 'just two glasses' rule and was clearly destined for another Uber ride home, which would mean an added headache the next morning of somehow getting the car back by 7 a.m. to get the kids to their various Saturday sports activities. This scenario was becoming increasingly familiar and one that I knew my husband would be quietly biting his tongue about, pretending it didn't bother him, while his disapproval radiated off him in waves. I'd been here many times before.

Later that night, after hurriedly putting the kids to bed and trying desperately to appear less drunk than I was, guzzling water and eating mints to hide the telltale whiffs of wine and Marlboro Lights (I only smoked when I drank but then I *was* drinking most nights these days), something really niggled at me.

Beccy's words were lingering in my mind and I couldn't stop thinking about them. *Do women of my age really have hobbies? Or any spare time to do things they love? How on earth do they make that happen?*

Truth be told, I didn't really do anything outside of running the kids around, working, keeping on top of the never-ending to-do list at home and exercising (which I would put in the category of 'justification for wine', rather than a hobby). And then, of course, drinking. Drinking, in fact, had become my one and only hobby. The only thing I did with any spare time, and the thing I did to counter the fact I barely even had any spare time. I was rarely without a glass in hand if it was past 5 p.m. and I was at home.

My evening wine was my solace at the end of the day. My reward. My line in the sand to signal to my overwhelmed and busy mind that it was now *my* time, and even if I had a million chores to still get through that evening, if I could do them with a wine in hand, it somehow made it more bearable. Pouring that first glass of wine was the moment I breathed a big sigh of relief that now I could finally do something for me after a day of doing everything for everyone else.

The only problem was that the wine wasn't working in the way it used to. I didn't get that same 'ahhhhhhhh' feeling after one glass anymore. That glass would be gone in the blink of an eye, barely touching the sides before I was pouring another in search of the release and switch-off that I so desperately craved but which was becoming more and more elusive. What had started as a glass most evenings had somehow morphed into a bottle (sometimes more) and I couldn't even pinpoint when or how that had happened.

Through the week I was increasingly feeling more tired, anxious, unmotivated and low in mood. I had a constant niggle in my belly, which then travelled up to my brain to whisper, 'Is this it? Is this really as good as life gets?' The monotony of work, kids and chores was broken only by the temporary high from a bottle of wine which then led to shit sleep, wretched hangovers and zero energy to do much more until it was time to drink again.

Nobody knew, but I'd started taking sleeping tablets every time I drank to avoid the inevitable 3 a.m. wake-up, which then left me even more groggy, slow and lethargic the following morning. Life felt like Groundhog Day, a never-ending treadmill of to-do lists with little time or space for anything else. I craved alcohol more and more to make these anxious, sad feelings go away, but this only led to more anxiety and more disrupted sleep. It was a vicious cycle.

On the outside, no one thought I had a problem. But inside, I was in turmoil. I'd turned 40 earlier that year and I was questioning my life, my future and myself in a way I never had before. It was confusing. Deep down I knew I was drinking at a level that was concerning, and the dependence on sleeping tablets also worried me, but I brushed those thoughts and fears aside because I didn't *want* to explore them any further. It was simply unthinkable to me to consider that alcohol was the problem or that I might need to change my drinking.

When my drinking romance ended

Alcohol had always featured prominently in my life since I began drinking in my teens. I put it down to the fact that I was a social person who loved a party and alcohol enhanced my mood. It was just a coincidence that I was *very* social and always seemed to be at a party! Through my 20s and 30s, I wore my heavy drinking as a badge of honour and gloated about my ability to endure twelve-hour benders, 'keeping up with the boys' and, after a few hours' sleep, continuing again the next day (sometimes never sleeping at all). To me, this stamina and tolerance for alcohol was something to be applauded and demonstrated with pride.

My drinking habits changed once I'd had children. This was at a time when some major events in my life collided: in 2010 I had my first baby and we made the decision to move to Australia. I left behind my success-ful and rewarding career as director of a recruitment firm, which I loved, my family, my core group of girlfriends, and the familiarity of everything I knew. Within a month of arriving in Perth I was pregnant again and soon had two kids under two, a husband who was working long hours to set up a new business, and although I was desperately trying to get out and about to make new friends, I found it hard. Much harder than I expected. When I did go back to work it was part-time in a job I didn't really enjoy. Those first couple of years in Perth were tough. I was homesick, I was lonely, I was sad and I was lost. In such a short time everything in my life had changed, from my career to my support group to the country I now called home. And so, I drank. I drank to numb those uncomfortable emotions. I drank to make myself feel better. I drank so I could pretend I loved my life in Australia but honestly, I didn't. I would never have said that out loud at the time but I was really struggling and alcohol, my trusty friend, popped up as the perfect solution to navigate all my inner sadness and confusion. For the first time, I was drinking more and more at home on my own. I was eyeing the clock to justify what time I could crack the first bottle. I can recall one day standing at the end of the driveway with my daughter in my arms and my son playing at my feet waiting for my husband to return from work while tears streamed down my face. I remember him taking the kids from me as I headed inside, poured a glass of wine and went out to the back deck to sit and drink until I didn't have to feel anymore.

Once I became more settled, made some gorgeous friends and set up my own recruitment business (which brought about its own stress), my drinking was less about trying to numb emotions and more a habit and a ritual to end the day. Although my new social life of BBQs, children's birthday parties, lunches and play dates was a far cry from the boozy, five-star restaurant dinners in London and the clubs of Ibiza, they still all involved wine. My drinking had adapted to my new lifestyle as a parent – I started earlier and finished earlier but I still drank.

Even once I secretly acknowledged to myself that my drinking was becoming problematic when I hit 40, I certainly wasn't thinking about the health risks of my alcohol use – I was actually pretty ignorant of them – but more how it was making me feel in terms of my weight, mental health and energy. Then a couple of things happened that were the turning point for me.

By 2017 my drinking had escalated. I was drinking in secret; I was more frequently craving alcohol on a Sunday morning after a particularly boozy Saturday night (it was the only way I knew how to make the hangover go away); and the 'rule' I set myself about never drinking on a Monday was being repeatedly broken. Did I acknowledge it was bad? No, I just ignored all those whispers; I didn't want to hear them. And so, as is the way with life, when whispers are ignored, the screams begin. The first turning point was at a friend's 40th birthday party in April of that year.

I was drunk before I even arrived, as was my way to 'get in the mood', a legacy carried on from university, when we were so skint we would drink as much as we could before we went out so we didn't have to spend as much on alcohol in the clubs. Once at the party, I downed shots like they were going out of fashion, and soon I was the only one on the dance floor happily swaying to 'Wonderwall' before I went outside for a fag. I knelt to put out my cigarette and toppled forward. Having no reflexes, I landed face-first on a concrete driveway. I split my lip, smashed my nose and there was blood everywhere. A friend took me home and put me to bed, trying not to wake my sleeping husband who had stayed home with the kids. I woke the next morning to my five-year-old daughter standing beside my bed, staring at me in confusion and asking, 'Mummy, what happened to your face?' As memories of the night before came flooding back with an awful stomach-sinking feeling, a little piece of me died inside.

The shame, the self-loathing, the regret. Later that day, in a world of pain, I sipped wine through a metal straw; my lips were too bruised to hold a glass to my mouth, but I had to find a way to get the alcohol into my system. It was inconceivable that I wouldn't drink. When I thought things couldn't get any worse, the following morning I went to my local pharmacy to ask what would make my smashed-up face heal as quickly as possible. While the pharmacist loaded me up with arnica and anti-inflammatory tablets, she also quietly slipped me a card, with a kind and compassionate look in her eye. The card had a helpline number for domestic violence. Tears stabbed at my eyes and began to stream down my face as I rushed outside to my car. I couldn't believe this woman thought my kind, would-never-hurt-a-fly husband could have done this to me. Another little piece of me died inside.

I would love to tell you from that moment I never drank again but that's simply not true. I carried on drinking and just three weeks later, there was another birthday, another huge drinking session that started at noon and ended at 3 a.m., leading to another early morning wake-up by a child.

This time it was my son, dressed in his cricket gear and holding his bat, gently shaking me awake to take him to cricket. It was just four hours from when I'd crashed into bed and, as I pulled myself upright, I just knew I couldn't drive. I knew I was still over the limit. And with that moment of truth came more shame and remorse. I couldn't take my son to the thing he loved most in the world because I was still drunk from the night before.

That Sunday, as I wasted another day lying on the sofa scrolling on my phone and counting down the hours until I could go back to bed, a post popped up in my running Facebook group (yep, I was still running half-marathons despite the drinking – it was my little way of again convincing myself I didn't have a problem with alcohol). The post was shared by a woman who said she'd just finished reading a book about alcohol which had completely changed her drinking, and how much faster and fitter she was for having stopped. That post hit me square in the eyes and I truly felt I'd seen it for a reason. I ordered the book and made a pledge to myself. I would do 21 days alcohol-free. I'd passed my tipping point and I knew I couldn't carry on the way I had been. I thought a 21-day 'reset' was all I needed to change my drinking, and so I began.

In all honesty, I didn't find it too hard. I was so ready for something to change and so sick of the hangovers and awful sleep that I truly embraced all that I gained in that initial 21 days: a clear head, improvement in my sleep and energy, being much more productive at work and no longer missing gym sessions or cancelling plans due to hangovers. I had a glimpse of the woman I was without alcohol – and I liked her! When I reached the 21 days I was feeling so much better that I saw no reason to return to drinking and decided to keep going. That 21 days turned into 100 and I'd never felt so clear, so calm, so energised, so happy. I felt like I'd finally had a glimpse of who I really was! But then a niggling voice started up again: 'You can't never drink again, Sarah, that would just be weird, you're Sarah the party girl!' And so I returned to drinking, believing that now I'd had a decent break, I would be able to tone it down and moderate. I would now be a 'normal' drinker.

Within a month I was back to drinking as much as before. But this time I had the knowledge of what life felt like without alcohol. And for the next two years I became stuck in the classic grey area drinking cycle of bingeing, abstaining for periods (a month, three months) then going back to drinking again, determined that this time I'd be able to moderate and be a 'normal' drinker. But it was just never the case and I always ended up back in the same place – drinking more than I intended, blacking out, breaking promises, my anxiety increasing. Finally, by April 2019 after a really booze-filled summer, I knew I had a decision to make: carry on drinking or stop for good. I finally accepted moderation was never going to work for me, no matter how hard I tried. I was mentally exhausted by the battle of constantly trying, and failing, to moderate. I knew in my soul I was done. I knew my life was better without alcohol. I knew I was a better mum, wife, friend and worker without alcohol. I knew *I* was better without alcohol. And I was and I am.

If anything I have written here resonates with you, then please know you are not alone. When I shared this very story in the women's online news site *Mamamia*, over 8000 women contacted me with the simple, startling message: 'You just told my story.'

What started for so many of us as drinking to socialise and have fun has morphed into our one and only tool to get through our days, and lives that sometimes feel like little more than one long, brutal, relentless to-do list. And let's not forget that everywhere we turn, we're seeing adverts that enforce the message that it's our right and reward to end our busy, stressful days with a glass of calming, relaxing wine. Is it any wonder that middle-aged women are drinking more than ever?

We are continually being sold the idea that alcohol is our 'reward' at the end of a busy day, something to look forward to, to ease our tired minds and bodies. And something that is completely justified. Memes and cards resound with messages such as 'Motherhood: Powered by love, fuelled by coffee, sustained by wine' and 'The most expensive part about having a kid is all the wine you have to drink'. And yet we've rarely paused to question this. Why would we? We recognise the problem (we are stressed, overwhelmed, too busy and too tired) and we have been sold the solution – alcohol. And so, we drink.

So many of the women I speak to would get honours degrees in multi-tasking. We are holding down busy jobs, raising kids, caring for elderly parents, running houses, cooking meals and feeling the social expectations and pressure to look good, do good and be good. And, for a moment, alcohol gives us that moment of quiet reprieve in a noisy, relentless world where it can feel like everyone wants a piece of us. We have very little time left over for anything else in our lives, and the thing about our evening drink is we can have it while ticking off the to-do list, as a way to make ourselves feel just a smidgen better among the feelings of chaos and being overwhelmed.

For many of us, we are silently aware that our drinking has increased beyond 'take it or leave it' levels. We may have a nagging voice that whispers we are drinking too much and sometimes we listen. We may take breaks from alcohol, complete a Feb Fast or Sober October, and this lulls us into a false sense of security. 'Well, I can't have a problem because I just took a month off.'

But the problem is often that, even if we've managed to stop for a month, we can't *stay* stopped. We often return to drinking with gusto, and then find we're drinking even more than before. Why is this? It's because we haven't considered the bigger problem.

Alcohol is not the problem here. Alcohol is the *solution* we have created for the initial problem, which is that we are overwhelmed, exhausted, lost, disillusioned and have no time for ourselves. Alcohol is also a solution to feeling lonely, bored and having no clear direction or focus on what we want to do with ourselves, our lives.

And when we do have spare time, we have no idea how to spend it doing something that brings us joy, because we don't know what that is, either. We have lost ourselves. Many of us are children of the 70s who started drinking in the late 80s or 90s and that's pretty much all we've done in our spare time. And alcohol has, for so many of us, provided a smokescreen of pretending (sometimes even to ourselves) that we are happy and satisfied with our lives. Yet as we get older, we're beginning to question what else we have in our lives, what makes us happy, what brings us joy, what we do outside of parenting, working, partnering, friending. What do we do for *us*? And we don't know the answers to these questions. And so, we drink.

Our social media images portray 'fun' and 'happy' as always being with a glass in hand at various social events, or relaxing somewhere with a cold glass of bubbles, '#andrelax'. But on the inside it's a different story; on the inside we feel lost, unfulfilled, confused and overwhelmed. We are like ducklings on the lake, looking calm and happy above the surface, but underneath our little feet are paddling a hundred miles an hour, barely struggling to keep from drowning. We feel like life is passing us by, the years are ticking on, and we've lost connection to who we are, our dreams and our joy. Even if we had an afternoon to ourselves, we wouldn't know how to spend it because it happens so rarely. We would most likely crack open a bottle to avoid those feelings of boredom, unfulfillment and slow-burning disappointment. In 2022 I posed a question to over 20,000 women on social media via my Instagram page and my Facebook community 'The Women's Wellbeing Collective'. The question was, 'Why do you drink?' The three top reasons were 'stress', 'boredom' and 'loneliness'. Just pause for a moment and let that sink in. Then consider, why the hell do we have a generation of women who are so bored, stressed and lonely that drinking alcohol is their only way to cope? More importantly, how do we change this?

The answer to both these questions lies in the fact that in our modern world so many of us have lost connection to ourselves, lost sight of what makes us happy, and exist in lives that barely allow for time to explore any hobbies and interests that bring authentic joy. We drink as a way to manage the stress and dull those uncomfortable emotions of loneliness and boredom.

But the good news is that we *can* make long-term change with our drinking, and create lives that are calm, interesting and fulfilling. And importantly, the key to making this change is to *add* something to our lives, not merely just take something away. If we just took alcohol out, and didn't add anything in its place, it's only going to leave a big, gaping void and then before we know it we're filling that void once again with buckets of chardonnay.

If we want to change our drinking, we *have* to look at all the other ways we can fill the hole that removing alcohol leaves. In so many ways, stopping drinking is the straightforward part. Staying sober and creating a life where we don't want or need to drink is at the true heart of the work I focus on with my clients – people just like you. You don't have to be an 'alcoholic' to decide to quit drinking and you don't have to be drinking a certain amount every night to decide to quit. You can simply decide you want to see who you are and what you could achieve in your life if you're not drinking.

This book is different to many of the wonderful sobriety books and stories out there. I'm not going to tell you how to *get* sober, but I'm going to share with you how to create a life where you don't even *want or need* the drink. So regardless of whether you are newly sober curious and testing the water, or you're two years sober and enjoying life but still feel like there's more for you to discover, I am here to show you how I did this and help you to do it, too.

Beyond Booze will support and guide you to dig deeper to explore your own personal relationship with alcohol and then offer tools and strategies for what you can add *in* to create long-term change with your drinking. To help with this, at the end of every chapter I've included some questions for you to consider in regard to your own experiences. You might like to write your responses in a journal or notebook for reference, or even use them as talking points with trusted friends. Reflecting on these questions is part of the 'work' that will help you add to your strategic toolbox for creating a rich, satisfying life without the desire for the numbing effects of alcohol.

Once I'd made the life-changing decision to remove alcohol back in 2019, it hit me that the focus shouldn't be on *just removing* alcohol. It was about so much more than that. I had to address the real problem behind my drinking: I had to look at *why* I was drinking in the first place. What purpose did alcohol serve in my life and what did I need to add *in* if I was taking alcohol *out*? If I could address those questions, I just knew that how I viewed alcohol would change.

What followed has been an incredible journey of discovering what I value in life and living in alignment with these values, discovering tools to manage my stress so I don't end every day exhausted, overwhelmed and anxious, exploring what I love to do with my spare time and who I actually am at my very core – my most authentic self. Because I had no idea. I'd spent nearly all my spare time for the preceding 28 years living very much on autopilot, drinking or recovering from drinking. And I suspect, if you're reading this, that you may not know – or remember – your most authentic self either. And that is exactly what we are going to discover through this book. This deep journey of self-discovery is where we will go, together. Because one thing I know to be true is that sobriety takes us back to our most authentic selves and allows us to step into the body and life of the person we were always meant to be.

Perhaps right now, reading this, it feels impossible to think you might ever reach this point of not relying on alcohol for all that it gives you. I know it did for me. I had used alcohol to celebrate, commiserate, numb emotions, enhance emotions and everything in between. Not having my trusty friend by my side felt like losing a limb. But I promise it *can* be fun and it *is* possible to create an incredible, interesting, fulfilling and contented life, alcohol-free. I'm living proof and so are thousands of other women across the globe.

Changing our drinking isn't a prison sentence: it isn't a 'less than' life. It's actually the gateway to an incredible life! It allows you to connect to yourself on such a deep level that you finally *know* yourself, what you love, what lights you up, how you want to spend your time and who you want to spend it with. You begin to trust yourself, champion yourself and finally, most importantly, to love yourself. And I cannot wait to help you get there. As one client described to me recently, it's like going from living in black and white to living in colour – we just have to know where to get the paint from.

So, consider this book your palette!

Much love,

Sarah Rusbatch

xxx

CHAPTER 1

ARE YOU A GREY AREA DRINKER TOO?

(Yes, there is such a thing)

Do you remember watching the TV show *Sex and the City*? If you're like me, then you probably idolised the main characters and all that they represented. I lapped up the sophistication that oozed from Carrie, Charlotte, Miranda and Samantha as they hopped from one rooftop bar to the next, Cosmopolitan in one hand, fag in the other. They shared stories of one-night stands, broken hearts and girlfriends who were the most important people in their life, all of which resonated with me so deeply at that stage.

Who was your favourite from the four? Me, I loved Samantha. I channelled her as I drank my way around the bars and clubs of London in the early 2000s (and okay, I probably picked up a bloke or two). Back then, my (rather large) love of alcohol was never a cause for concern. I was young, free and single! Did I worry what the future would hold as my friends and

I screamed 'girl power' and downed shots of tequila? No. What about when we doused our hangovers with Sunday-morning bloody Marys? Definitely not. It was the era when we were told that women could have it all and our role models were women drinking with carefree abandon as they sought independence and equality.

What we watched on TV, in movies or saw on billboards and posters was the same consistent message – we *needed* alcohol to have fun, make new friends, attract the opposite sex, be an empowered woman and experience all that life had to offer. Quite simply, without alcohol, life was boring.

It never occurred to any of us *not* to drink. We never even considered it. It was our rite of passage into adulthood and drinking bottles of Lambrusco (urgh!) while applying our makeup and listening to the Spice Girls was happening in bedrooms across the globe.

Yet somewhere along the way, those innocent boozy nights morphed into solo drinking at home, behind closed doors. This is when our drinking progressed from 'so much *fun*' to 'just *one* to relax us while we make dinner, get the kids sorted, empty the dishwasher and run the bath … *oops, there goes the bottle!*'

Our responsibilities increased with the taking on of mortgages, partners, jobs, perhaps a kid or two. And, like so many women I speak to, with that shift in age and responsibility came the change in our drinking habits (more home-based solo drinking, less partying) which neatly coincided with the messages we were now receiving about alcohol in adverts and product placement in TV shows.

It was in the 1990s that the major alcohol companies began segregating their markets and targeting different sectors, including deliberate campaigns aimed at women, specifically very young women, with the introduction of 'alcopops', also known as 'alcohol with training wheels'.

This advertising segregation has continued ever since, with differing campaigns aimed accordingly at different age groups of women through their various life stages. Messages promoting alcohol as being for fun and partying aimed at teens and young women morphed into messages of alcohol being sophisticated and powerful for women in their 30s, which progressed to alcohol as a reward, a relaxant and something we 'deserve' at the end of a busy day in our 40s and 50s. And this hasn't been without its repercussions.

We have now normalised something that really isn't normal – it's not normal or healthy to drink every night of the week or to get absolutely plastered every weekend. It's not normal or healthy to rely on alcohol as our only crutch to navigate the stress, feelings of overwhelm, loneliness and boredom we are experiencing in our lives. But we are acting as if it's the most normal thing in the world.

The problem with pink messaging

We now live in a society that promotes alcohol as the common solution to all the struggles modern women face (our mothers certainly weren't exposed to the alcohol messaging that we are today). And the messaging is often so subtle or subliminal we don't even recognise it's happening. How many times have we been watching a police drama on TV and seen a female detective walk in the door after a long, hard day at work and immediately pour herself a glass of wine? Or seen for yourself the specific focus on young mums, a demographic already exhausted, vulnerable and overwhelmed, being sent blatant messages that they 'need' wine to be a parent via Mother's Day cards that read, 'Dear Mum, thanks for passing me the wine gene', and Babygros with slogans across the front saying things like, 'I whine so Mum drinks wine.'

The alcohol companies are always finding new and strategic avenues to sell their products to us in ways we often don't even realise. Due to the recent restrictions on alcohol advertising, and a growing awareness around alcohol advertising through social media, advertisers are facing increasing pressure to create ads that tap into our emotions on every level. A 2019 article titled 'Experiential Marketing for Alcohol Brands' concludes: 'Creating a successful marketing campaign for an alcohol brand is now a matter of activating experience at every touch point.'

The alcohol brands are trying to make us 'feel' something when we see adverts for their product and, in most cases where women are concerned, this is the promise we will feel relaxed, connected and rewarded. Not coincidentally, there has been an increase in 'pink' drinks over the last couple of decades, mainly due to the fact they are so easy to promote. In a 2019 research article conducted by the Public Health Advocacy Institute of Western Australia, Curtin University, titled 'The Instagrammability of Pink Drinks', the findings were conclusive in that:

> It is evident that the alcohol industry in Australia is designing and promoting alcohol products specifically for women. The themes identified in this report highlight that products designed to appeal to women are often pink and palatable, use imagery that is highly likely to appeal to young women, and include health-related claims such as low sugar, low calorie, and natural ingredients.

And it's working, because more women are drinking at binge-drinking levels than ever before. We believe we 'deserve' that drink at the end of the day. 'Hell yes, we do!' has said pretty much every woman across the world at 5 p.m. when the witching hour arrives and we can crack open that first bottle. Spy on any mother's WhatsApp group chat about the relentless juggle of parenting, working, managing the house and all that it involves and across the world the advice is the same: 'Go pour yourself a wine and just relax.' (I know because I was the one advising this day in, day out!)

The more we're told it's 'normal' to drink at the end of a stressful day (and show me a woman who isn't experiencing some sort of stress at this time), the more we've allowed it to creep in (and creep up – because who stops at one?). Our evening drink is about as regular as brushing our teeth – but have we ever stopped to question the impact it's having on our health? Canada has! In fact, in early 2023 the Canadian government dropped their alcohol recommendations to no more than two alcoholic drinks a week with a recommendation of zero on the back of a report by the Canadian Centre on Substance Use and Addiction. The report concluded that no amount of alcohol is safe and having any more than two drinks a week is risky.

Which now poses the questions for the rest of the world: *What is an acceptable level of alcohol consumption? What is considered okay? And when does it stop being okay?*

The reasons we are normalising heavy drinking

I often reflect on why I never paused, not once, to question the health impact of the amount I was drinking. I've concluded that there were two main reasons. I suspect they both may resonate with you.

1. Information on the physical risks specifically related to women's vulnerabilities when it comes to metabolising alcohol wasn't readily shared or available.

2. The relentless marketing and advertising of alcohol, along with contemporary social expectations of alcohol being present and consumed at nearly all social gatherings, normalised my everyday drinking.

I thought I was just like most of the women around me and it was completely normal to end every day with a glass or two (or more) of wine … because I *was* like most others! It has become normal and, in fact, promoted, in our society to drink in this way. But it's *not* normal and it's not healthy and it holds us back from living our best lives, but we don't even know that because we've never taken a long enough break from drinking to get a glimpse of the difference. (Pregnancy doesn't count – I don't know about you, but I was a hormonal mess during both my pregnancies so that didn't give me any glimpse of what an energised, sober, happy life would be!)

And because everyone around us is often drinking in a similar way, we rarely pause to reflect on the role alcohol plays in our life or whether it's adding or taking anything away. As I have said previously, it never even occurred to me to consider a life without alcohol. I was just so utterly brainwashed by the relentless cultural messaging that alcohol *added* to my life. Not to mention that, for the most part, I also loved getting pissed. Even though it was robbing me of my sleep, energy, clarity of mind, motivation, self-connection and self-esteem, it didn't occur to me to stop because I sought that oblivion and feeling of escape that alcohol offered. I believed a life without alcohol wasn't worth living and I thought a night spent getting as drunk as possible and not remembering how I got home was the most fun a middle-aged woman could have in a life that consisted of working, raising kids, running a busy household and very little spare time.

I was so wrong.

AN ALCOHOL-CENTRIC SOCIETY

Tell someone you've quit smoking and I can guarantee the immediate response will be: 'Good on you! Well done! So proud of you!' Tell someone you've quit drinking and wait for the awkward silence to fall, or perhaps the odd uttering of 'Oh don't be so boring, just have one.' I was at a dinner party recently where a woman I'd never met before went to fill up my glass with wine. 'Oh, no thanks,' I said. 'I don't drink.' She paused, a look of confusion on her face before asking, completely seriously, 'Why? Are you an alcoholic?' When did someone choosing not to drink alcohol make them an alcoholic? When did we all fall for the story that we need alcohol to have fun, socialise and connect, and we would only choose not to drink if we had a problem with it?

Let's consider for a moment where alcohol is present in our lives. It's everywhere! At every major event, celebration and commiseration (ever been to a wedding or funeral that didn't serve booze? Hell, I've been offered wine after a yoga class, a half marathon and at 10 a.m. at a kids' birthday party). It's the only drug we have to justify *not* taking and its use is normalised in nearly every Western culture. Yet we can't ignore the fact that a neatly packaged, sparkling pink liquid with aromas of cherries and butterflies is a Group 1 carcinogen.

In fact, in a 2023 World Health Organization report titled 'No level of alcohol consumption is safe for our health', it says:

> Alcohol is a toxic, psychoactive, and dependence-producing substance and has been classified as a Group 1 carcinogen by the International Agency for Research on Cancer decades ago – this is the highest risk group, which also includes asbestos, radiation and tobacco.

Yet we glamorise it, promote it, encourage each other to consume it and dish out peer pressure when someone says they don't want it (yep, guilty as charged). The more we do this and the more we rely on it to manage our stress and feelings of overwhelm, the longer we stay stuck on the merry-go-round of drinking, hangovers, disillusionment, exhaustion and anxiety.

The fact alcohol is expected, accepted and is celebrated is hugely problematic in society.

There's no denying it's hard to quit drinking in an alcohol-centric society. That's why I applaud every single person I meet who makes the decision to go against the societal norms and conditioning and dare to want more for themselves. It's particularly hard when we are constantly bombarded with incessant marketing that depicts beautiful people cracking open refreshingly staged drinks on a hot summer's day.

Ever seen an advertisement that depicts the following morning after a big night out – head down the toilet, tears streaming down the face, scrapes on elbows and knees? I think not. Alcohol companies and advertising want us to see only one aspect of their product and they will throw everything at it to ensure that's what we believe.

In fact, in the US alone, alcohol advertising spending in 2023 was set to hit US\$7.7 billion. In Australia, the most recent study (which was still twenty years ago) shows this spend to be in excess of \$220 million and in the UK, if everyone drank the recommended units of alcohol each week (14 units or a bottle and a half of wine per week), the alcohol industry would lose approximately 13 billion pounds (around AU\$26 billion) a year. Let that sink in … if we drank in moderation the alcohol industry could go bust! While the alcohol companies might share messages to 'drink responsibly' or 'drink in moderation', in my opinion this is just lip service – their spend on alcohol advertising is significant and targeted, with the sole purpose of getting us to buy and drink more.

The problem with this targeted and relentless messaging of normalising and justification of regular alcohol use is that we simply stay stuck in the disillusionment and constant exhaustion it causes and nothing changes. In our ever-busy worlds, alcohol is sold as the easy way out, and who doesn't want that? And remember, this marketing is aimed at women of *all* ages, which hasn't been without its consequences.

The specific marketing directed at young women in the UK from the early 90s coincided with an increase in the diagnosis of liver cirrhosis and liver cancer in women in their 20s. David Jernigan, director of the Center on Alcohol Marketing and Youth at Johns Hopkins University, said of this statistic in a BBC interview: 'The cancer doctors in the UK are blown away, they have never seen anything like it.'

And unsurprisingly for middle-aged women, binge-drinking and alcohol use disorder are only increasing. Coincidence? I think not! For context, alcohol use disorder is defined as a medical condition whereby a person is unable to stop drinking, even though they may want to, and has negative physical, mental and relationship consequences. It includes the stages of drinking that some people refer to as alcohol abuse, alcohol addiction or, as we often call it, 'alcoholism', and can be classified as mild, moderate or severe. In terms of amounts of alcohol consumed, it is generally classed as eight or more standard drinks (or 12 units) a week. The Australian Bureau of Statistics classes binge-drinking as four or more standard drinks on one occasion, which for many of us drinking at home would be two large self-pours of wine. I could easily have consumed two large glasses of wine (which would likely be four units) on a light night and have exceeded eight units by Wednesday.

I felt disheartened when I considered all these facts. Due to the aggressive marketing and society's normalisation and acceptance of drinking, most of us have fallen into the category of alcohol use disorder without even realising it – it's simply what we've been doing to get by. I felt like I'd simply been a pawn in some huge conspiracy to get me to drink more, with little regard for the consequences to my health, and I'd fallen for it hook, line and sinker. The truth was, I had. We all have. And through sharing our lives on social media, we have all (unknowingly) been playing a part in exacerbating this problem.

Our kids are being exposed to this from a young age, too. Last Mother's Day, a well-known nightwear store in Australia had a mannequin in its window wearing PJs with red wine glasses all over them, holding a cask of red wine (*yes!* a cask of wine!) in one hand and a wine glass in the other. I shudder to think how many little girls saw that mannequin and, like us, were influenced by the subliminal message that 'mums need wine'.

We have a generation of stressed, overwhelmed, exhausted and anxious women who never need telling twice they 'deserve' that glass of wine at the end of the day. And boy, have the alcohol companies capitalised on that message, with pink gins and beautiful bottles, not to mention the school parents' cheese-and-wine nights or gin-tasting events, and memes that fly around everywhere you look that say things like, 'I choose my kids' school friends based on how much their mother drinks' and 'I heard that if you drink every day, you're an alcoholic. That's why I only drink at night.'

We're juggling more than ever and feeling increasingly stressed. We are expected to raise grounded, resilient children, care for elderly parents, maintain friendships, keep fit, help at the school P&C, be a porn star in the bedroom, Nigella in the kitchen and Arianna Huffington in the boardroom. The pressure is *on*. And boy, did I feel it. Do you, too?

Gabor Maté, one of the world's leading specialists in addiction, as well as parenting, said in a podcast interview with parenting expert Zoe Blaskey: 'This is the hardest time to be a mother since the Second World War.' So many of us are living separately from our extended families without the support and connection our ancestors enjoyed; we are often working full-time in paid work and then the night shift starts once we hit home. COVID-19 blurred the lines even more between work and home life, and any previous work–life balance boundaries we had went out the window. We have little spare time and feel a generous serving of guilt if we even attempt to do something for ourselves. And so, we drink. And boy, do we drink!

In fact, as revealed on the BBC Radio *Woman's Hour* show titled 'The Feminisation of Alcohol Marketing', the stats are hard-hitting. A 2017 US study found that 'alcohol use disorder among females skyrocketed 83 per cent between 2002 and 2013'. And in Australia, a study in the 2022 *Drug and Alcohol Review* showed one in five Australian women are drinking at binge-drinking levels. (Remember, binge-drinking is more than four standard drinks at any one time, and alcohol use disorder is described as eight or more drinks a week. I was drinking that some nights!)

WOMEN'S PHYSICAL VULNERABILITIES

There are numerous reasons why the increase in alcohol use among women is so concerning, and none more so than the way alcohol affects women's bodies. The fact is that a woman's physiology simply does not and cannot process alcohol in the same way that a man's does, which makes us much more vulnerable to the health risks caused by alcohol. There are three core reasons for this:

1. Women are more deficient in the key metabolising enzyme alcohol dehydrogenase (ADH) which helps the body break down and eliminate alcohol, meaning a higher amount of alcohol enters our bloodstream. This explains why cognitive deficits, heart issues and liver disease occur earlier in women than men with significantly shorter exposure to alcohol.

2. Men have a higher percentage of body water. As alcohol dissolves in water, alcohol is more concentrated in a female body than a male body. The higher the concentration of alcohol in a body, the greater the damage it can cause.

3. Fluctuating hormones can impact how intoxicated women become. Depending on the time of the month and how high our oestrogen is at any given point, we may get more drunk even if we drink the same amount of alcohol. This explains why some nights we are more impacted by alcohol than others. It's important we know this. It's also important our daughters know this so they understand that at different times of the month they may become more drunk than they normally would, may be quicker to lose control of their faculties and may expose themselves to riskier situations.

There are many other health risks too, in regard to the effects of alcohol on women's bodies. The Alcohol and Drug Foundation of Australia reported a study that one in ten breast cancer diagnoses in Australia is linked to alcohol use. (And yet, I bet like me, most of the cancer fundraisers you've been invited to have free-flowing champagne. Ever been to a cancer fundraiser that has given you a free fag as you walk in the door? No, I didn't think so, yet both have the same carcinogenic risk.)

Further afield, the World Health Organization stated in 2021 that breast cancer has become the most common cancer globally. More than two million new cases were estimated in 2020, and about 100,000 of these were attributable to alcohol consumption. It concluded: 'Alcohol is one of the

WHAT IS SOBRIETY TO YOU?

'The most beautiful relief. It's like breathing in fresh, cool air after being stuck down in a dark, stuffy bunker for what felt like eternity.'
KIRSTEN

'Falling in love with myself, one day at a time, more and more each day.'
KATIE

'Waking up from a bad dream.' SARAH

'Freedom!' SUZANNE

biggest risk factors for breast cancer. Simply reducing alcohol consumption can greatly reduce the risks.'

When I interviewed Kathryn Elliott, a breast cancer survivor and public speaker, she said:

> Drinking any amount of alcohol increases your breast cancer risk. Many studies have looked at drinking and breast cancer risk and they've all found that the risk of breast cancer increases as alcohol consumption increases. Compared to women who don't drink at all, women who have three alcoholic drinks per week have a 15 per cent higher risk of breast cancer.
>
> In Australia, awareness is low with only one in five women reporting to know that drinking alcohol is a risk factor for breast cancer.

The Cancer Council of Australia also states that alcohol is related to the development of six other cancers: mouth, throat, oesophagus, stomach, bowel and liver. And you are more than six times at risk of developing oral cancer if you are a drinker.

On top of this, alcohol has now been linked to many other diseases which negatively impact health including high blood pressure, stroke, heart diseases, liver disease, weakening of the immune system, learning and memory problems like dementia, leaky gut and a strong link to anxiety and depression. Dr Helena Popovic, a leading authority on improving brain function, recently devoted an entire chapter in her latest book on dementia prevention, *Can Adventure Prevent Dementia?*, on the impact of alcohol on the body and brain, which shocked me to the core. It included the facts that alcohol accelerates ageing and takes years off our lives by shortening our telomeres (the protective caps on the ends of our chromosomes); four standard drinks a week triples our chances of developing dementia; people who develop face flushing after consuming even small amounts of alcohol regularly are ten times more likely to develop oesophageal cancer than people who do not get red in the face, and one night of binge-drinking reduces the ability to perform complex memory tasks for up to four days. She also states that alcohol is linked to 60 acute and chronic diseases and that the World Health Organization states that there are 8000 alcohol-related deaths a day. To put this into context, COVID-19 was responsible for 6000 a day and yet off-licences and bottle shops were listed as essential services during pandemic lockdowns. And despite all this, we still consider our evening drink as a 'treat', a 'reward' and a suitable gift for any adult birthday party we attend!

As alcohol causes us so much harm, I can't write a book about building a life without alcohol without referring to this at least once.

To be clear, I am not anti-alcohol in terms of advocating for prohibition. I've had many wonderful, memorable (as well as not so memorable!) experiences with a drink in hand. And there are many for whom alcohol is not a problem and causes no significant harm to their lives, their mental or physical wellbeing, how they parent or their relationships. I have several friends who happily drink without any kind of issue with alcohol, and there is zero judgement from me.

But what I *am* about is sharing relevant and factual information on what alcohol is doing to our beautiful bodies so we can all make an informed decision on when and how much we drink. And I am about supporting those who want to make a change, for whom drinking has started taking more than it's giving, but don't know *how* to make that change when we live in a world where alcohol is everywhere we turn.

Because I do know that there *is* another way to live life, and that you don't have to stay stuck in a pattern of misery and regret if you feel alcohol is no longer serving you. And you don't have to hit rock bottom to decide to quit or take a break from alcohol. It's not about reaching a 'number' that tells you it's time – it's more about a feeling.

If you feel in any way that alcohol is taking more than it's giving, whether you drink a glass a night or a bottle a night, you have full permission to take a break. If you've ever questioned your relationship with alcohol or the role it has in your life, it might be a sign that you are ready to make a change, whatever that looks like. For many of us it starts as a little voice that's whispering through the fog of the booze or the hangover, 'This isn't good, this isn't working, this isn't the way forward.' Looking back, I can see I had many of those moments but I simply ignored them for as long as I could, because I didn't want to listen. I wasn't ready to.

There is a famous saying by Albert Einstein: 'Insanity is doing the same thing over and over and expecting a different result.' And for many of us, that's what we're doing with this continuous cycle of drinking, then pledging the next morning not to drink that night, only to find ourselves at 5 p.m. pouring that wine on autopilot and beating ourselves up for drinking when we said we wouldn't. Or countering our drinking with hardcore gym sessions, diets of smoothies and protein, and taking every supplement under the sun, yet still drinking like a fish and wondering why we don't lose weight or feel better (yep, story of my life!).

But if this is how you feel, please don't blame yourself. As well as the constant marketing and promotion of alcohol, we also have to remember that it's super addictive! And, as with any addictive substance, we build tolerance to it, so we eventually need more and more. Remember when one drink used to be enough and now it doesn't even register? What starts for so many of us as a glass at the end of a stressful day 'to take the edge off' quickly increases to two glasses and then, before we know it, we are drinking a bottle most nights, and/or perhaps opening a second.

You might be reading this and thinking, 'Oh, but I'm not addicted to alcohol', because you don't drink every day or you take breaks from it. But here's the thing. We can be addicted but not drink every day. We can be addicted but not drink in the morning. Alcohol is addictive and if we've been using it regularly and consistently over years it only makes sense we do become addicted to it. We just don't want to admit it because for most of us, 'addiction' feels like a dirty word and something shrouded in shame.

There is no shame in becoming addicted to one of the most addictive substances in the world.

What is addiction?

Let's consider for a moment the definition of addiction. Addiction expert Gabor Maté describes it as manifesting in 'any behaviour a person finds temporary pleasure or relief in, and therefore craves, suffers negative consequences from and has trouble giving up'.

Tick, tick, tick! I found temporary pleasure in my drinking; I craved it, it made me feel terrible and yet I had trouble giving it up. But I still would never have said I was addicted to it. Until I dove deeper into understanding what addiction really is.

You see, the crazy thing about our modern world is that we have created a society that deems some substances and behaviours acceptable to be 'addicted' to – sugar, caffeine, social media, online shopping – and even jokes about or mentions them with pride ('I'm feeling bad and I'm off for some retail therapy' or 'I can't possibly start my day without coffee, don't even speak to me until I've had my morning hit'), whereas others are looked down upon, to be kept secret and hidden.

Alcohol falls into that second category for many of us. We've been led to believe that only the 'weak' become addicted to alcohol. Yet alcohol is promoted everywhere and we are always expected to partake, but if we develop a 'problem', that's our fault. The fact is, we have known for some time that women become addicted to alcohol quicker than men. This view was prevalent even back in the 1930s when the Alcoholics Anonymous fellowship's 'Big Book' was first released, which stated that women become addicted to alcohol quicker than men do and that, 'Potential female alcoholics often turn into the real thing and are gone beyond recall in a few years.' I wonder if this information was taken into account when the alcohol industry began relentlessly targeting women to increase their sales? Somehow, I doubt it.

Our culture has done nothing to help with the stigma around alcohol addiction. I would guess that for most of us, our knowledge of alcohol addiction is associated with images seen on TV and in movies of dingy church basements where people scurry inside to whisper in shame and remorse, 'Hi, I'm Sarah and I'm an alcoholic.' We have to stop stereotyping alcohol addiction! And we have to offer people help at any stage of alcohol use disorder. I recently spoke to a client who was turned away from a drug and alcohol rehab facility in Perth because she wasn't drinking 'enough'. For context, she was drinking one to two bottles of wine a night but this wasn't deemed enough to make use of their services and she was simply told to 'cut down'.

I didn't, and would never have, described myself as an alcoholic. But, like many in a similar stage of drinking, I did have a problem with alcohol. The labelling, however, is problematic and it's the stereotyping that prevents so many from getting the help they need.

In fact, in Catherine Gray's book, *Sunshine Warm Sober*, she refers to Dr Nick Sheron, a liver specialist in the UK who said only one in three of his patients with alcohol-related cirrhosis have 'severe alcohol dependency'.

The other two thirds are 'heavy social drinkers'. Yet both groups had the same significant liver damage. This is where, in my opinion, labels become problematic and prevent people getting help early enough.

One of the ironies of society's complex and contradictory attitude to alcohol is that you're ridiculed for not consuming it, yet frowned upon if you become addicted to it. 'Drink responsibly' says the alcohol industry yet it certainly doesn't suit anyone in the Big Alcohol companies for us to do this. In fact, as discussed earlier, if everyone in the UK drank responsibly, the alcohol industry there would lose a lot of money.

According to a study carried out by David Nutt, Director of the Neuropsychopharmacology Unit in the Division of Brain Sciences at Imperial College, London, alcohol is the fifth most addictive substance in the world (after heroin, cocaine, nicotine and barbiturates) and the only one that is freely available to purchase in any amount at pretty much any time of day. The remaining four substances are either illegal (heroin and cocaine), only available on prescription in limited amounts (barbiturates) or carry major health warnings and advertising of it has been banned (tobacco). Yet alcohol continues to be promoted, applauded and expected at almost every social gathering in the Western world.

SHADES OF GREY

While I never considered myself an 'alcoholic', it really resonated with me when I came across the term 'grey area drinking'. It made complete sense that this was where I sat (and where the women I work with sit). Grey area drinking is a term coined by Jolene Park, my coach and mentor, back in 2016 when she pioneered the grey area drinking movement. Her 2017 TEDx talk of the same name has been viewed across the globe by hundreds of thousands (I highly recommend watching it if you haven't already). The term describes people who consume more than a moderate amount of alcohol but don't meet the criteria for actual dependence. It's the 'grey area' between every-now-and-then drinking and rock-bottom drinking.

Although grey area drinkers might not drink every day or have a drink first thing in the morning (the widely perceived view of an alcoholic), they are likely to be preoccupied with alcohol and have difficulty giving it up.

Grey area drinkers are likely to be in the middle of the scale of alcohol use disorder. I describe it like this: imagine a person's drinking as being on a scale of one to ten. One is someone who rarely drinks, maybe has a champagne at a wedding once a year. Ten is someone at the severe end of alcohol use disorder who needs medical support to withdraw from alcohol (because alcohol is one of only three substances that we can die withdrawing from). Grey area drinkers, in my view, are people who sit between a four and an eight on that scale. Most don't view themselves as in need of help but they do acknowledge their alcohol use is having a negative impact on their life in some way: physically, mentally or both. Grey area drinkers have passed the point of 'take it or leave it' drinking and are using alcohol for something else – as a reward, a relaxant, for confidence, to switch off or to numb themselves from their emotions. Despite their regular use, they often haven't hit rock bottom, although most find there have been several small rock-bottom moments along the way, but nothing as big as losing a home, job or relationship as a result of their drinking.

Below is a list of some of the signs of grey area drinking to help you determine if you fall into this category (or previously have fallen, if you've already removed alcohol).

EXERCISE: CHECK YOURSELF

Let's check your vitals for signs that you're a grey area drinker.

☐ You make 'rules' about your drinking (how many, how often, what type of drink, what time of day, what day of the week) but you often break them. People who don't have a problem with alcohol don't make rules around their drinking.

☐ You secretly worry about your drinking and often regret what you said or did when you drank.

☐ You take breaks from alcohol. You may not drink every day, but you find it hard to stay 'stopped' and keep returning to old habits.

☐ You aren't always honest about how much you drink.

☐ On the outside, no one questions your drinking (you're high functioning) and it certainly doesn't appear you have a 'problem', but for you, it feels like a problem and is something you worry about more and more.

☐ You live with a constant internal 'chatter' about alcohol, always negotiating with yourself when you will drink next.

☐ You're a long way from rock bottom, but alcohol feels like it's robbing you of life. You're starting to feel like it's taking more than it's giving, but you don't know what to do next.

If you've checked off any of the above, it's a sure sign you lie in the grey area drinking zone.

When we take a moment to reflect, we can get real with the impact our alcohol use is having on us. Because let's not ignore the fact that, as well as impacting our physical health, alcohol is also having a huge impact on other important areas of our lives. I see it time and time again. Alcohol keeps our lives small. And in particular, it keeps *us* small.

We all desire amazing, fulfilling lives. But in so many ways, alcohol prevents us from achieving this. Alcohol stunts our growth and our potential and yet we don't even know it, as we've never taken a long enough break to see the difference! We stay stuck in a pattern of unfulfilled dreams, unmet needs and disillusionment with our lives and so we continually turn to the bottle to soothe our battered souls. However, all we are doing is preventing change and blocking getting what we actually want – which, for the most part, is joy, energy, fulfilment, presence, contentment and vitality. Who can go on to achieve all they want in life if they are constantly hungover, tired, anxious and unmotivated – living, at best, a five-out-of-ten life?

Is it hard to break the cycle of what is, for many of us, decades of drinking? Yes, it is. Any kind of change is hard at the start. But it's not hard forever.

Choose your hard

Before we move on to discussing all the tools, strategies and resources that this book has to offer, I do want to share with you something that I wish had been shared with me earlier in my own journey of removing alcohol. Which is that *how hard it is at the start is not how hard it is forever.* Not drinking in the first few weeks or sometimes months can feel like a full-time job and it can be exhausting! I remember having to plan, organise and structure my life to minimise cravings, avoid triggers and prevent awkward questions I didn't feel ready to answer. This was on top of dealing with the daily cravings for alcohol. But here's the thing – it's not like this forever.

Quitting alcohol is hard but gets easier;
staying drinking is hard too, but gets harder.

I can promise you it will get easier. If you've picked up this book and you want to change or have already changed your drinking, you will know by now that staying drinking is hard, too. Waking with feelings of shame and remorse, and not remembering what you did the night before is hard. Feeling like you're living half a life in terms of energy, motivation and potential is hard. Feeling exhausted, withdrawn and anxious is hard. Feeling like you're not being the mum, wife or friend you want to be is hard. Living with regret is hard.

A problem that many people encounter when first starting to change their drinking habits is thinking that how hard it feels at the beginning, is how hard it's going to feel forever. In the early days, staying sober is all consuming and every moment is spent simply trying not to drink. So they throw in the towel and pick up a drink again, going back to where they were initially. Clare Pooley's book, *The Sober Diaries,* has a brilliant analogy of the early part of sobriety being like an obstacle course where the beginning is full of really difficult obstacles, placed really close together but, over time, they start to spread out and the course becomes an easy, flat walk with just the occasional hurdle, and eventually the obstacles disappear altogether (I can't tell you the last time I had a craving for alcohol – well over three years ago). But most people never get to the easy part; they just keep repeating the hardest part. Let this book be your guide to never needing to do the hard part again. You are going to be armed with all the tools and resources to ensure you have added so much *in* that you won't want or need alcohol.

I remember this overwhelming feeling that I had more to offer the world, that I had more potential, but I just wasn't using it. And I see this time and time again: when women take a break from alcohol, *everything* starts to open up. It's like watching a butterfly emerge from a cocoon, as women start to grow and spread their wings, stand up for themselves with a newfound sober confidence and clarity, and start reaching for and achieving goals that had previously been hangover pipe dreams. It's simply incredible to witness.

AND THERE IS HOPE!

I'm sure by now, you're probably thinking, 'Okay Sarah, I get it, but what do I *actually* do? I know I want to change my drinking and create a better life but what's the process to achieving this?' If you're anything like me then it's possible you've taken time off here and there, read all the memoirs on sobriety and yet still find yourself returning to the same drinking patterns that you know in your heart aren't serving you any longer but feel powerless to control. Or perhaps you've quit drinking but you're still not reaping the benefits of a fulfilling life without alcohol.

Let's understand why.

First, and most importantly, if we aren't addressing the root cause of why we're drinking so much in the first place, we aren't going to be successful in removing alcohol from our lives. This is because if alcohol has become a crutch or coping strategy in some form (which for nearly all grey area drinkers it has) we first need to identify what alcohol has become a crutch *for*, so we can find another way of coping. We have to be curious about looking at our life, our patterns, our triggers and our behaviours so we can make positive, supportive and appropriate change where it's needed.

Second, when it comes to removing alcohol, we can't just remove it and then carry on living life exactly as we were before and expect to be happy. This is the biggest mistake I see people making.

We have to *do the work of sobriety* too. We have to look at what we are adding *in* when we are taking alcohol *out*.

This means learning to regulate our overworked nervous system and find new ways to manage stress and feelings of overwhelm so we don't get to the end of each day exhausted, depleted, emotional and automatically reach for the wine. It's about getting to know our own nervous system to discover what soothes us, and then doing more of that. (On a sidenote, I didn't even know what my nervous system *was* in the beginning and perhaps you don't either. Don't worry, by the end of this book you are going to know your nervous system inside out and will have learnt many ways to support it.)

We need to review our social life, where we hang out at the weekends and with whom, so we aren't doing the same things with the same people but just not drinking. Instead, we need to change it up and try new activities, meet new people with similar interests and begin to look at our spare time through a completely different lens.

We can begin to heal any past hurts and traumas which we may not have addressed for years (hello, school-girl bullying memories we've shoved down deep in the hope that if it's buried it will never affect us again – nope, doesn't work like that). When we remove alcohol it's normal for past traumas and experiences that we haven't dealt with (and only ignored by numbing with alcohol) to come rushing to the surface for us to finally process and release (more on this later).

We have to learn to set personal boundaries (and hell, I didn't even know what a boundary *was* when I first got sober) so that we can say *no* to others and *yes* to ourselves. This will free up time, energy and mental headspace to allow us to create a life we love, doing things we love, with people we love.

We have to get to know ourselves, to create a connection with our most authentic selves, something that is impossible to do when we are drinking most nights. We can't have a deep self-connection when we're half-pissed or battling a hangover every day.

And we have to discover what we love doing for fun, interest, enjoyment and inspiration. Once we do, we won't ever find ourselves bored, lonely and unfulfilled with that gaping hole inside us screaming to be filled with wine.

Ultimately, we have to create a more interesting, fulfilling and purposeful life by getting to know our most authentic selves. This is the fun bit! We get to explore who the hell we are without alcohol. We get to experiment with activities and experiences to discover what really lights us up. We get to discover, at whatever age we are, what we want to do for fun. Because as it turns out, what we loved doing aged 27 may not be what we love doing aged 47. And yet most of us are still trying to do the same thing and wondering why we don't enjoy it anymore. We have to embrace this new season of our lives with curiosity, interest and compassion. When you do, I promise, it's so worth the effort. In fact, it's magical.

So many of my clients look at me with fear, bewilderment and sadness in their eyes when I ask them, 'What do you love doing for fun outside of drinking? What are your hobbies, what fulfills you?' They don't have a clue (and once, nor did I). But we can commit to being open and exploring this with curiosity and interest.

Because hear me out. This is your one precious life. Your only life. And this is your moment to decide to start creating your best version of it, instead of trying to numb yourself from it or simply 'waiting' for something to change without making the active decision to change it yourself. Decide now! Commit to different. Commit to *you*!

> **It's finally time to stop numbing yourself from life,
> and start living it. Are you ready?**

Before we move on to all the practical tools, strategies and resources, it's important to acknowledge that, for many of us, alcohol has been masking something or has become a solution for something. And we need to identify what that is before we can start implementing the tools. We will look at this next.

SOBER ACTION STEPS

- ☐ Start noticing product placement of alcohol and/or advertising of alcohol around you. Once you open your eyes to this you will be amazed!

- ☐ Reflect on messages you've picked up on or bought into where alcohol is concerned, often subconsciously.

- ☐ Consider the grey area drinking checklist and ask yourself: on a scale of one to ten, where do you sit?

- ☐ Commit to the tools, tips and strategies I will be sharing throughout this book. Recognise that to be different we have to do different, and I'm going to show you how.

JODY

I was always the party girl. From the time I started drinking when I was sixteen and went out using my sister's ID, it was just 'normal' to drink, one drink after another.

I had a corporate job in my late 20s to early 30s, which involved a lot of entertaining with a company credit card. Several times a week I was wining and dining clients at the city's finest restaurants. I didn't consider alcohol an issue. It was part of who I was and it was fun to drink ... until it wasn't.

From my mid-40s I started to question my relationship with alcohol and feel that my behaviour at times was quite cringe-worthy and embarrassing when I drank to excess. I became loud and argumentative, particularly with my four sons and husband. I was also very active on social media when I had a wine glass in hand. I would read some of the rubbish I posted and think how ridiculous it sounded in the light of day.

I had an argument with my husband one night after drinking a bottle of wine. Something snapped and I physically attacked him and called him vile names. I was totally mortified and he was shocked and disappointed in me. That was really the first time we had a conversation about my drinking.

I stopped drinking at home for a bit then resumed, hiding it from him initially, and then gradually reintroduced it back into my daily life.

Looking back, I had a couple of drunk episodes over a few years in my late 40s to early 50s including tripping over and splitting my chin, accidentally putting nail hardener in my eyes instead of eye drops, and many days of feeling horrendously hungover, shaky, anxious and downright miserable.

A couple of years ago, we had a dinner with extended family including my elderly mum. At this point I was drinking well over a bottle of wine per day. I had been drinking all afternoon on an empty stomach and was already a bottle of wine down before we went out. At dinner I was nasty to my mum and when we got home my husband told me how horrid I had been.

It was at that point I turned around to him and said, 'I am not drinking anymore.' I recall him saying, 'What, tonight?' And I replied, 'No, I mean never.' I stopped that night and never had another one.

I filled in my evenings with things I enjoyed such as reading, taking walks and bubble baths. I rejoined the gym and also cleaned up my diet. It didn't take long before I not only felt better physically and mentally, but I looked better. I lost the bloat from alcohol, my eyes became whiter and brighter, my skin glowed and I lost 10 kilograms.

Being alcohol-free has given me freedom in the sense that I no longer hide bottles, credit card statements and hangovers. I connect with people on a deeper level and am a more considerate, patient person.

I am a work in progress in terms of checking off some bucket list items that I have added since becoming sober, and I still need to prioritise myself a little more to achieve some of these goals, but I will get there.

CHAPTER 2

THE UNCOMFORTABLE TRUTH

Peeling off the booze mask

Can you remember the first time you got drunk? Or what it was like when you first started drinking? I can.

At age thirteen, in 1989, we had moved from Scotland to England, I had a thick Scottish accent, a terrible perm and felt like I stuck out like a sore thumb in my new, strict all-girls school where everyone seemed sportier, cooler and prettier than me. I struggled to fit in. My first experience of getting pissed (at age fourteen in the local park with a group of my school mates) gave me a glimpse of what alcohol could offer me. Suddenly I didn't feel like the outsider; I felt like I finally belonged and was part of 'the gang'. Getting drunk with a group of girls became my way of feeling accepted, liked, perhaps even loved. It was my way of connecting. I loved it.

What followed was years of using alcohol to form friendships, create more connections and fast-track feelings of love. From fresher's week at university to Friday night drinks in my London graduate job to back-packing bars around the world, I learnt alcohol was a way to make friends and fit in quickly. 'You're my best friend,' screamed drunkenly at me in some pub toilet by a random girl I'd met only hours earlier, was music to my ears.

What started with Diamond White cider and ridiculous concoctions from my parents' drinks cabinet (Southern Comfort, Malibu, sherry, Martini, vodka or Baileys, topped with a bit of Coke – I can feel the vomit in my mouth as I share this with you) consumed in the park or roller rink with all the local kids, soon progressed to pints of cider at the student union bar and bottles of bubbles in fancy cocktail bars around London, then buckets of Bintang beer in Thailand and, finally, rosé over lunch while the kids played. The locations and the drinks changed, but the reason I was drinking never did: to gain acceptance, connection and friendship. To fit in. And then later to numb myself, switch off and unwind. I wonder what comes up for you as you read this? What's your drinking story?

For some, alcohol offered a tool to gain confidence in social settings. I've watched the quietest of people take centrestage in a karaoke bar after a bottle of prosecco. And while you may wonder if that is even a problem – who doesn't need a bit of Dutch courage before belting out 'I will survive' – it does become one if we are doing it so much that we don't even know who we really are without booze, because we've created a persona based on our drunken alter ego. If we're naturally quite shy and we drink for confidence, are people ever really getting to know our authentic selves?

I cannot tell you how many women discover in sobriety that they actually aren't the life and soul of the party, that they are actually introverts who are happiest in smaller groups, having more authentic conversations with people they know and trust. Do we ever even really know who we are, or what we value, if we're constantly using booze to mask shyness, fit in or change our personality in some way?

Of course, using alcohol as a social lubricant is only one of numerous ways women use alcohol – many also use it to numb emotions, relieve stress and as a pick-me-up at the end of a busy day. However, what is common to most drinkers is the fact that they are using alcohol for *something*. (We will cover this in more detail soon.)

From magic to medicine to misery

In the sober world, we talk about the three Ms of alcohol use to describe the three stages of drinking that many of us move through as our drinking progresses. Alcohol often starts as magic, moves on to become medicine and then morphs into misery.

1. MAGIC

For most of us, the first few years of drinking are 'magic'. This stage can last for years. It's 90 per cent fun and 10 per cent hangover to begin with, so it feels like the benefits far outweigh the negatives – nothing that a coffee, a couple of Panadols and a bacon sandwich can't fix.

When we are in the magic phase, we continue to reinforce the belief that alcohol equals fun. We are out socialising with our friends, laughing, dancing and dating. So often our friends continue to feed this narrative by declaring things like 'Oh you're so fun when you drink.'

Many people with alcohol use disorder (which you might remember is defined as more than eight drinks per week) look back on the magic phase and realise this was actually when the problems started. Because it provided *so much* magic. Some people discover alcohol and it really doesn't do much for them; they can take it or leave it and often this is their attitude to alcohol their entire lives. For others, right from their very first experience with alcohol, they feel it gives them something that really seems like magic. ('Oh yes!' I scream as I write this. You, too?)

And it's those of us who experience the big hit of 'magic' who are more vulnerable to becoming grey area drinkers (or develop more severe alcohol use disorder) because who doesn't want to keep going back for more if it's giving so much? Alcohol will never have the same pull or desire for someone who doesn't experience that magic hit when they consume it.

2. MEDICINE

This is when our alcohol use morphs from something that is used only to enhance a great night into something that becomes a solution to a problem, aka 'medicine'.

The problem might be that we are stressed, lonely, bored, angry, tired, sad or disappointed and we learn that picking up a drink makes that uncomfortable emotion disappear, albeit temporarily. We not only use alcohol to have a good time but also as a cure, a remedy. Medicine.

Again, we can stay in this stage for years and not even be aware that our drinking has morphed from magic to medicine. We are drinking on autopilot, rarely questioning how much or why or if it's even impacting us negatively. Most women I work with are in this stage.

3. MISERY

This is when we are getting so little from alcohol, yet our desire and need for it remains high. Our physical health is deteriorating, our mental wellbeing is decreasing and we are living with more dependence on alcohol. We've passed the point where we notice what we get from it – we just know we *need* it.

Our hangovers are lasting longer, and we don't get the same high from that first drink, but we just keep on drinking because we don't know any other way. Our alcohol use has passed the point of being a choice; it's become a way of life and one that we don't necessarily enjoy, but feel powerless to stop.

LET'S REFLECT

Before we move on, it's important to have an honest conversation with ourselves. Below are two question that might help you work out where you are right now regarding your drinking.

1. What stage would you say you are at currently, or were before you quit drinking?

2. Can you identify when you switched from one stage to another?

What mask are you wearing?

While I was using alcohol initially to create friendships and form connections, it later became my tool to avoid sitting with big emotions of sadness, anger, loneliness and stress. I didn't have any other tools to process these uncomfortable feelings so I simply drank them away. As I write this, I immediately think of a song by UK singer/songwriter Raye, called 'Escapism', which has a line that catches my attention time and time again: 'I don't wanna feel, so I stick to sippin'.'

Learning where we're at with alcohol and what it is masking or hiding is essential in our journey to a happy, booze-free life.

Alcohol is a coping strategy for avoiding so many uncomfortable emotions or big events in life. For grey area drinkers, alcohol nearly always shows up as an escape route of some kind. We're not using alcohol to enhance a good mood or to enjoy a glass of red with our steak – it's more than that. We drink to become numb. The problem is that our emotions are there for a reason. If we don't allow them to have their space and voice, but simply distract ourselves from them, they come back to bite us on the bum, big time. One of my favourite quotes on this topic is from an ancient text known as the Gospel of Thomas. It says:

If you bring forth what is within you, what you bring forth will save you.

If you do not bring forth what is within you, it will destroy you.

We have to let ourselves feel our feelings because if we don't, they can destroy us. When all we do is ignore or suppress our feelings (as so many of us are doing with alcohol), I believe they only become stronger and build up inside us until we explode in some way. Ever heard the old saying, 'If you never heal from the pain that hurt you, you'll bleed on the people who didn't cut you'?

The issue for so many of us is that we've never been taught how to sit with uncomfortable emotions or process them in a productive and healthy way as children. I certainly was never taught this at school or at home. Were you? I couldn't even have named an emotion beyond happy, sad or angry and yet, as a highly sensitive child, I was feeling these big emotions all the time.

This is why, when we discover tools that soothe us in the moment, we are drawn to them. Anything that takes us out of ourselves, even temporarily, works to keep our emotions pushed down inside. Alcohol is the perfect example here, but there's also drugs, overworking, overexercising, people pleasing, food, scrolling on social media, gambling or excessive shopping. From a young age most of us are taught that distraction is the solution to pain or discomfort. 'Oh, you've hurt your knee, let's rub it better and get you an ice cream!' or 'You feel sad because you had an argument with your bestie? Come and have a chocolate and make it all better.' Sound familiar? This isn't to criticise our parents in any way; they were often doing what was modelled to them and, in the short term, distraction *does* work to soothe us if we feel pain or sadness. But it also means we never develop a robust, healthy toolkit of resources to navigate through life's pain and hardship. And when we discover alcohol, it can quickly become our medicine, and often our only solution.

I can remember as a thirteen-year-old coming home from my new school, still trying to make friends, feeling lonely and insecure, and heading straight for the bread bin. I would eat crumpet after crumpet layered thick with butter and chocolate spread as a way to distract and soothe myself from those difficult emotions. I didn't tell anyone how I was feeling. On the outside I was 'fine' but on the inside I was anything but. I self-soothed with food, particularly sweet and fatty food, and this developed in later years into alcohol use and then recreational drugs as ways of escaping any uncomfortable emotion, especially loneliness. In his book *Recovery: Freedom from our addictions*, author Russell Brand describes sugar as the gateway drug. It was for him and it was for me too. What about you?

> **Alcohol is not the problem, it's the 'solution' to the problem.**
> **It is a mask, a way of *numbing* ourselves and *avoiding* what's**
> **really going on. To remove the need for alcohol we need**
> **to address the underlying problem.**

One of the first tasks in our journey towards changing our drinking habits and behaviours is discovering *what* emotions alcohol has been masking and/ or what it has become the solution *to*. Then we can address those emotions in a healthy way so we remove the need for alcohol at all. Many of us have been drinking for so long we don't even know why we're doing it and think all we have to do is remove alcohol and everything will be fine. That's simply not the case because alcohol was never the initial problem.

The seven main masks

Honestly, I am yet to meet any woman who identifies as a grey area drinker for whom alcohol isn't masking *something* or working as medicine in some way. As Dr Pamela Stewart, a psychiatrist at the Centre for Addiction and Mental Health in Canada, says, 'Typically, men drink to heighten positive feelings or socialise. Women are more likely than men to drink to get rid of negative feelings.'

I've worked with senior partners of law firms using alcohol to mask chronic anxiety and imposter syndrome, wives deeply unhappy in their marriages using alcohol to numb their feelings of discontentment, and teachers using booze to switch off at the end of an insanely stressful, overwhelming day. The circumstances may vary but the reasons are often the same – lack of confidence, escapism, distraction, oblivion and avoidance.

The most common emotions or feelings that I see alcohol helping us to mask, either earlier in life or in our present day, include:

1. **Loneliness** – Perhaps you were like me and often felt you didn't quite fit in and were always on the periphery in some way, but when you discovered alcohol it felt like you were let into the 'inner circle' and accepted. Maybe this carried on into your adult years and became your tool for making friends and avoiding being alone. Or perhaps your kids have left home, or you've struggled to make new friends in adulthood, or your social life has become smaller and you feel an increasing sense of loneliness and disconnection.

2. **Sadness** – No one likes feeling sad. But in most cases, it's an appropriate emotional response to an event that has happened. Showing this emotion makes us vulnerable so we tend to mask it and ignore it. So few of us have ever learnt to sit with sadness but instead always try to minimise and distract ourselves from it. It's a major reason for drinking.

3. **Shyness / social anxiety** – Perhaps you struggle in big groups and worry about what to say or that anything you do say will sound silly, until you drink and become more confident and feel funnier. This might often be reinforced by friends who appear to like you more when you have had a drink, and make you feel that you're dull or boring without alcohol. (I can't tell you how many people this is the case for.)

4. **Stress** – Ever used alcohol to unwind, relax, switch off and escape your own head for a while? It's a brief reprieve from the never-ending pressure and to-do list that makes you feel like you are going to explode! With that first drink you start to feel that pressure disappear, albeit temporarily (something we'll cover in detail soon).

5. **Anger** – What a difficult emotion to sit with! Maybe you've had an argument with your boss or partner, and you just don't know what to do with all the big, angry emotions flooding your body. Alcohol offers a way out, a way to shut down all the adrenaline that has been generated (because alcohol is a depressant, after all). Anger is a big-energy emotion that most of us have not been taught how to deal with, so we stifle it through drinking.

6. **Boredom** – One of the more common reasons for drinking. So often we are busy and yet also mentally bored and unfulfilled. We're rushing around every day but nothing we're doing is satisfying us or lighting up our soul. And when we do have spare time, we've become so disconnected from ourselves, we don't even know what to do with it. Alcohol actually dumbs down our brain and makes boring things appear more interesting so it's a pretty quick way to alleviate this issue. But seriously – who wants a life where they have to dumb down their brain to make boring things more interesting? What kind of a life is that? (There is an alternative, I promise.)

7. **Hormones** – For women, extreme premenstrual tension (PMT) symptoms can really increase the desire to drink. I know many women who are fine for three weeks of the month and don't even think too much about alcohol and then the week before their period

all hell breaks loose. Their mood changes, their cravings increase and they feel powerless against picking up the bottle. I even know of women with active alcohol addiction who have been treated in rehab centres using hormone replacement therapy to reduce alcohol cravings – that is how strong a role our hormones can play in our desire to drink.

LET'S REFLECT

- ☐ How many of the seven masks did you just tick off in your head?

- ☐ Do you drink to give yourself confidence and courage in big groups? Do you drink to fit in and be 'accepted' by your peers?

- ☐ Do you drink to distract yourself from and make yourself numb to feelings of sadness or shame?

- ☐ Is alcohol your go-to strategy any time you feel stressed or overwhelmed?

- ☐ Do you notice your cravings for alcohol increase at certain times of the month?

Only when we know *why* we are drinking can we start to create long-term, sustainable change.

The case of the dry drunk

Before we go on, it's important at this point to address what it means to *not* do this deeper self-inquiry work.

In sober communities across the world, we refer to a 'dry drunk' as someone who takes a break from booze (or removes it completely) but doesn't do any of the deeper work that is really required to address *why* they were drinking in the first place, and which ultimately is the gateway to creating long-term change. In most cases, they keep everything else in their lives the same except for not picking up a drink, or they swap their alcohol use for something else as a way to numb themselves, such as food, exercise or online shopping.

Often a dry drunk will take a break from alcohol but simply cross off the days until the necessary self-imposed time of abstinence has ended. When they return to drinking (sometimes even after really extended periods of time, such as months or years), they believe they will now be able to drink in moderation and with control. They are often surprised and confused when they can't.

This can be the cycle for many grey area drinkers: they take breaks but their drinking quickly returns to the levels it was at before. (This was certainly the case for me.) That's because we don't do the deeper work to address the issue of why we are drinking in the first place. And if we don't do the deeper work, the reasons we were drinking in the first place are still there, so it makes sense we are going to pick up our drinking exactly where we left off, no matter how much time has passed.

Some people ask me: 'If I do the work on myself in sobriety, then wouldn't I be able to return to alcohol and no longer use it in a dysfunctional way?' I reply: 'Well, if you do the work properly, you won't even want or need to return to alcohol in any way whatsoever!'

Perhaps you're recognising this pattern in yourself. How many times have you taken a break from booze, only to discover that the moment you return to it, your drinking continues at the same level, or perhaps gets even worse – like suddenly you're playing catch-up! Dry July, Feb Fast, Sober October or any of the other increasingly popular months in the alcohol-free calendar are, no doubt, to be applauded for the way they get so many of us to abstain from drinking for a period of time. However, if you are a grey area drinker, then they do little to create any long-term change (especially if all we are doing is crossing off the days and celebrating with a huge bender at the end).

The sad fact is that I used to decline social invitations during those months of short-term abstinence from alcohol because, in my mind, there was simply no point in going and mingling with people if I couldn't have an alcoholic drink in my hand (I'm actually cringing at myself as I type this but it's honestly where my thoughts were, and shows the grip that alcohol had on me).

The first time I quit alcohol, I didn't do any work on myself. I just crossed off the days. Although I did appreciate waking happy and refreshed, as time went by, and the novel feeling of never being hungover, always sleeping well and having mental clarity wore off, I became complacent.

The hangover-free life had become my new normal, but as I hadn't done any of the deeper work (which we will cover in the next chapters), I listened to the wine witch when she once again reared her ugly head and started whispering, 'Oh come on, you weren't *that* bad, you could just have a couple with your friends or on special occasions – what's the worst that could happen?'

And I believed her. This is a classic case of 'fading affect bias', something that happens to nearly all of us. William Porter, in his book *Alcohol Explained*, describes this well when he writes: 'Fading affect bias essentially describes the process whereby good memories persist longer than bad ones ... where we tend to view events in the past in a more positive light as time passes.'

This means as time passes, our memories of the negative impacts of alcohol begin to fade and instead we only remember and focus on the positives, such as that cold glass of wine on a Sunday afternoon at the beach, or that gin and tonic at sunset. Our brain doesn't remember the 3 a.m. wake-ups, the anxiety, the wretchedness as we suffer through most of the day hungover, counting down the hours until it's over. Our brain only remembers the positive. (A lot of us wouldn't go on to have a second child if that wasn't the case, right?)

YES, BUT WHAT ABOUT MODERATION?

Is moderation even possible? This is something I get asked all the time. For me, there were so many times I listened to that little voice when it promised that '*this* time you will be able to moderate' and '*this* time it will be different'. But it just never was. And so every time I returned to alcohol after a break, I was always surprised when I couldn't moderate and it never was just one glass (always a bottle instead). I couldn't understand why.

To put this into context, let's consider your drinking on a scale of one to ten. If you consider yourself currently a six out of ten and then you take a break from alcohol, no matter how long for, when you pick up a drink again it's only a matter of time until you get back to six. And I mean a very short time. I was back to my normal levels the third time I drank after 100 days off. For some it's the first time they pick up a drink after three years sober. And remember, at six out of ten, we can still have a level of addiction to alcohol. We don't have to be at ten to be addicted.

Professor of Psychology Dr Judith Grisel says: 'There is no good evidence that shows you can go back to moderate use after being addicted.' And Professor David Nutt, who specialises in addiction as well as neuropsychopharmacology says: 'Your brain learns addiction just as it learns to ride a bike, so your brain will remember.'

I've seen people take five years off from drinking and immediately return to where they were before. And sadly, I've heard of people who have died because of this: although their brains picked right back up to where they were before, their bodies could no longer tolerate such huge levels of alcohol.

So many of us think that moderation is the ultimate goal. But for many of us, it's completely impossible. And it can be the ultimate prison sentence for those who achieve it. Because even if they do manage to moderate, they don't *want* to moderate. They want to drink with abandon and with no regard for consequences. To moderate they are using every ounce of willpower and mental energy to stick to the prescribed number they have dictated as being acceptable, but it's extremely tiring and takes up so much headspace.

It make sense to me that when we stop trying to moderate and choose to completely remove alcohol, we free up so much headspace. We are no longer living with the internal chatter and negotiation of 'Will I drink tonight? I said I wouldn't drink tonight but I really fancy one, maybe I can have one and leave it at that? But if I did want two I could, because I don't have to be at work tomorrow til late so I can have a lie in, and if I do have two then I definitely won't drink the next night, etc, etc.' Moderation is exhausting! It takes up so much mental energy. Imagine how you would feel and who you could be if you put that extra mental energy to good use!

When I conduct discovery calls with clients who reach out to me for help, the form I ask them to fill out ahead of our calls asks the question: 'What do you want to change about your drinking?' Over 90 per cent respond by saying they want to be moderate drinkers; they want to be able to enjoy a glass of wine every now and then and not always overindulge in the way they are currently.

I often ask if they were ever moderate drinkers in the past. Most reply 'Never' or 'Maybe in my first few months of drinking, but then it became more.' What they want from me is to make them the type of drinker they've never, ever been. And I'm not a bloody magician!

There is a well-known saying in the sober world: you can turn a cucumber into a pickle but you can't turn a pickle into a cucumber!

Hardly anyone says they just never want to drink alcohol ever again. And the reason most want to drink moderately is because we are constantly being sold the message that a life without alcohol is a 'less than' life, that we 'should' be able to moderate a highly addictive substance and it's up to us to 'drink responsibly'. This messaging puts all the onus on the drinker and none on the companies who are selling this highly addictive substance.

As I've said, if you've tried moderation and it didn't work for you, it's not your fault. For some of us it's that our brain dopamine pathways get lit up more by alcohol than the next person (more on this in the next chapter), for others it's a coping strategy that is so deeply embedded it's become a way of life. For many it's both. And for nearly everyone I have encountered who has passed the point of being a 'take it or leave it' drinker – what I would consider a five or more on that one-to-ten scale – moderation simply isn't an option.

For me, there was no doubt about it: I *loved* getting pissed. I sought oblivion. In fact, I craved it. I never wanted just one or two. I mean – who even are these people who are happy and content with just the one? I lived by well-known rock musician Florence Welch's statement: 'If I enjoy my drinking, I can't control it and if I control my drinking, I don't enjoy it.'

For me, having to control my drinking was the greatest punishment there was. Going out for dinner with friends and having a waiter pouring the wine only when he saw fit was my idea of hell. I would sit watching the others' glasses, willing them to drink quicker so we could all get a top up, silently praying the waiter would give me just a bit more. I would feel the panic rising that the bottle would be emptied and I wouldn't have had enough. On those nights I often went home and continued drinking alone simply to reach the level of oblivion that the night hadn't offered. I felt cheated until I reached that point. But when my drinking reached the stage where it started taking way more than it was giving and was impacting me both physically and mentally, I had to make a decision: was it going to be none or was I going to carry on as I was? Because I knew the third option of moderation simply wasn't possible. Once I finally came to realise that moderation would never work for me, I made the decision it was going to be none. And with that decision came absolute freedom.

Once I had made the decision to quit for good, I also knew that if I wanted to succeed (which I truly did) then I had to do it differently than all the times in the past where I had taken a break and then returned to drinking with the aim of moderating. I was so sick and tired of trying (and failing) to moderate. I had to ask myself, what *was* success for me in this scenario?

I realised success was not simply 'not drinking' through sheer willpower. In actual fact, success was *not even wanting* to drink. Not craving it, not thinking about it and not idolising it. Which is where I am right now and have been for some time. As I write this, I can tell you hand on heart that there is not a fibre of my being that wants to pick up a drink. When I say this in podcast and radio interviews, I am often asked: 'How do you reach that point, when alcohol has played such a key part of your life for so long?'

And the answer is by doing *the work*, and I'm going to show you exactly what I mean by that in the following chapters. But it's important to explore some of the additional factors that lead to us developing grey area drinking habits first.

Model behaviour

Something to consider when we reflect on our own drinking is how alcohol was role-modelled to us as kids. This is not to be judgemental but instead curious about where and how your first beliefs around alcohol were formed. Were your first beliefs around alcohol positive? Did your parents have lots of parties where there was always alcohol present? Did you watch your mum having a glass to unwind after a long day, or your dad enjoying a beer when watching the footy? This isn't about questioning whether our parents had a problem with booze or saying they did anything wrong if they did have a drink; it is about recognising the subliminal messaging we received from such a young age.

Alcohol was prevalent in my home growing up and I can now understand it clearly did influence me in a couple of ways. The first is that my parents were really social and often had raucous dinner parties where the wine was flowing, the adults were merry and the laughter was loud. My earliest recollection of this was on 'Robbie Burns night', a traditional night in the Scottish calendar to eat haggis, drink whisky and recite Scottish poetry. I remember drunken men in kilts staggering around giggling, and shrieking laughter coming from the dining room. My seven-year-old self hid behind the door and looked on, enthralled and wistful as I watched the adults dancing, singing and, oh my, having so much fun! I couldn't wait to be old enough to attend events like this – and of course they would involve alcohol, it never occurred to me that they wouldn't. From my observation point, alcohol equalled fun. The neural pathways were forming at that young age (as I'm sure they were for so many of us).

As I started to grow older, I saw how alcohol could be used to soothe all kinds of uncomfortable emotions. I remember overhearing my parents have an argument and then watching Dad head straight over to the drinks cabinet to pour himself a whisky. It didn't register at the time as 'Oh, look at Dad numbing his emotions'. But it clearly registered on some subconscious level. Because when I had an argument with my first serious boyfriend, guess what I did? Yep, I headed straight for that same drinks cabinet, grabbed that glass and poured a stiff drink (monkey see, monkey do!). I still remember the burning (but not unpleasant) sensation, the hard liquor hitting my throat and making its way down to my stomach, a feeling of warmth settling in, a numbness …

But as I mentioned earlier, this isn't about *blaming* our parents. They were only doing what was 'normal' back in the 70s and 80s, as alcohol was being promoted and marketed to them like it is to us. Drinking was something to have fun with and something everyone did as an adult to unwind, socialise and connect at weekends after a long working week. It was normal and expected. At this point for so many of our parents, alcohol was providing 'magic' and it wasn't problematic. But we were still subliminally receiving the message at a very young age that alcohol equals fun as an adult. As Paul Dillon, the director and founder of Drug and Alcohol Research and Training Australia, says: 'Children are influenced by their parents' drinking behaviour.'

I also want to acknowledge here that some children do grow up in homes where their parents' or guardians' alcohol use is not 'fun' but instead severe, damaging and detrimental to the child's life. This can also have an incredible impact on a child's future drinking habits. I see this usually go one of two ways – the child never drinks alcohol because they have seen the impact it's had, or they go on to develop alcohol use disorder as that's what has been modelled to them. I will talk more about this later.

The fact is that for many of us right now, our drinking has escalated, perhaps not where we would be described as an alcoholic, but to the point where we are often picking up a drink in response to a difficult emotion or uncomfortable experience. To be clear, life will always have issues and we will always experience uncomfortable emotions, but when we hide or distract ourselves from those issues, we never learn ways to sit with those uncomfortable feelings and process them in a healthy way. We never learn to 'sit in the shit' as my friend Ash Butterss, host of the recovery podcast 'Behind the smile with Ash Butterss', calls it.

Unless we learn to deal with and process our pain and our uncomfortable emotions, we will never build resilience to deal with life's issues as they arise and so we just drink more and more – another vicious cycle.

We say in the sober world that when you quit drinking you resort back to the emotional age that you were when you started drinking, because you've never learnt healthy ways to process emotions. Think about it – how old were you when you started drinking? That means there's a hell of a lot of teenagers wandering around in adult bodies with shitloads of growing up to do!

If I had my way, in every school across the world, we would spend more time teaching the next generation how to sit with uncomfortable emotions – *not* avoid them. Because this is a skill we are lacking, and yet is so necessary.

But we can teach ourselves new tools to navigate uncomfortable emotions and in turn, we can teach this to the next generation.

In fact, one of my proudest moments as a parent occurred recently with my eleven-year-old daughter, after a really busy and stressful day, which included back-to-back zoom calls, a car that wouldn't start, and not a single moment to myself to simply breathe. Just before I jumped onto my last call of the day at 7 p.m., I said to my daughter, 'Oh I'm really feeling it today, Mum's at the end of her stress ladder.' When I finished the call she gently took me by the hand, whispering, 'Come with me.' She led me into the bathroom where she had prepared a Zen-like sanctuary, with candles, soft music, an inviting bubble bath and my favourite essential oils. And you know what? In that moment, I was so grateful that I'd quit booze because I can assure you, her response a few years ago would have been to wait outside my door with a wine glass in hand. I also felt so incredibly proud that I had modelled to her true self-care and that she had picked up on it. It reinforces that our kids are always watching and noticing what we do.

In Ann Dowsett Johnston's brilliant book, *Drink*, she says that daughters of alcoholic mothers are much more likely to develop problematic drinking habits themselves because they've never had healthy self-care modelled to them. I don't think you need to have severe alcohol use disorder to relate to this. And I don't think you have to be a parent.

Remember, when you make changes with your own drinking you are also impacting the pathways and alcohol associations that any young people around you will have. I received a note from a client's son recently. She had just hit six months sober. His note said simply: 'Thank you, Sarah, for giving me my mum back.' Never underestimate the impact of not drinking on those around you, particularly the younger generation.

Think about how drinking was role-modelled to you ...
Then pause and think, how are you also role-
modelling it to others?

SOBRIETY FEELS LIKE ...

'Opening the door to the magic of
the rest of my life.'

SONJA

'The path to being fully present in
life and enjoying the best mental and
physical wellbeing.'

ELIZABETH

'The freedom to live and feel ALL of
my emotions. I am able to be truly
present for my child, my family, my
friends and myself.'

MIRANDA

LET'S REFLECT

☐ Do your kids ever see you socialise without alcohol?

☐ Do your kids see you drink most nights?

☐ Do you model healthy tools for managing stress outside of alcohol?

This isn't about shaming you, but about getting real with understanding that changing our own drinking now changes the drinking of the next generation.

The past drives success in the present

While I am not (and have never professed to be) a psychologist, I have been connected to enough sober people and supported thousands on their own journey to sobriety to know that often there are factors from our past that are driving our desire to drink. I won't focus on this in too much detail, as there are so many more incredible resources on this topic that can provide more support and information than I can (and I have listed these at the back of this book), but I feel it's important to mention as part of this chapter, where we are exploring why we may be drinking at a dysfunctional level and identify that these reasons may have started at quite a young age.

Several of my clients discover, with the clarity of being alcohol-free, that they have been shoving down and numbing emotions for a big part of their lives.

A word that many of us baulk at is 'trauma'. Historically, we have been led to believe that trauma is a word used only to describe major, catastrophic, often life-threatening events such as living or fighting in a war zone, physical or sexual abuse, or the death of a loved one. However, I have learnt through extensive reading and from my own experience of therapy that while these events describe 'Big T' trauma, there is also something known as 'Little T' trauma.

Little T traumas are events or experiences that are non-threatening and can (and often do) go unrecognised and unprocessed but still cause distress, particularly in childhood. If they weren't processed effectively at the time, they stay with us and can drive addictive behaviours and dependencies (more on this in Chapter 4).

Little T traumas are vast and varied and can include growing up in a home where the parents were unhappy with a lot of tension and arguing, dealing with a sick or alcoholic parent without support, bullying, feeling excluded, lack of attention from parents (emotional childhood neglect), emotional abuse, death of a beloved pet, public humiliation or being made to feel ashamed by teachers, coaches or parents, or constantly moving house and having to make new friends. These are just a few examples. These events, I would argue, can cause *more* distress than first thought because they are so often ignored and not given the attention they require to enable us to process them healthily when they happened and move on. Often Little T traumas are not even shared with primary caregivers or, if they are, are brushed under the carpet or belittled.

In the now famous 1995 Adverse Childhood Experience (ACE) study, medical doctors and researchers Vincent Fellitti and Robert Anda highlighted traumatic events in a child's life that led to a higher risk of developing mental, physical and social problems as an adult. As well as the more singular, majorly traumatic events (Big T) of abuse and violence, the list includes some Little T traumas, including violence in the community or school. From the study we now know that an individual who experiences four or more Little T events in this study is seven times more likely to identify as having alcohol use disorder. Gabor Maté made a very famous statement about exploring the reason behind any kind of addiction. He said, 'The first question is not why the addiction but why the pain?'

It's therefore important to acknowledge that this deeper self-inquiry work of exploring what may have occurred in our younger years that led us to become grey area drinkers may require professional help. In fact, I would argue that it *must* include professional help in order to safely explore events that we may have kept hidden or suppressed for years. And there is absolutely no shame in doing this. In fact, I actively encourage it. Working with my therapist, Chris, who I began seeing in 2019, has been the most profound and life-changing experience for me and the greatest act of self-care I have ever shown myself.

Our opportunity to heal

We are so fortunate to live in an era where there are so many resources available to support us to heal and learn how to navigate and process difficult emotions in a healthy way. These include podcasts, books, TED talks, websites, webinars and courses. (I have included some at the back of this book that have had a profound impact on me.) Little (if any) of this was available to our parents' generation. In Chapter 4 I share some tools and resources that have hugely benefitted me learning how to manage and process my emotions, and not fly off the handle or reach for a drink every time I face adversity. I truly believe there's no greater gift you can give yourself than the gift of your own healing and happiness. And there is no greater gift you can give the people you love most in your life, including your children, than your own healing so you can show up as your most authentic, true self and in turn, model to them what that actually looks like.

Once we've begun the journey of healing, we can also begin the journey of exploring what we need to add *in* when we take alcohol *out*. That's exactly what we'll get into next. The remainder of this book will explore the steps to creating a life where you no longer want or need to drink, because you've started to address the root cause of why you're drinking in the first place. Hooray!

EXERCISE: GET REAL

Now is a great time to grab a pen and journal and reflect on *why* you drink. The following questions may help you.

1. What role did alcohol have in your house growing up? Do you notice any unconscious beliefs you may have created around alcohol at a young age?

2. How old were you when you started drinking? Can you remember how it made you feel and what you got from it?

3. Can you recall times when you have used or craved alcohol in a specific moment where you felt uncomfortable? What was the emotion you were trying to avoid?

4. What are your beliefs around alcohol? Do you believe it relaxes you? Makes you more fun? Gives you confidence? What do you get from drinking? And is what you believe actually true?

5. What can you identify as the gaps in your life that alcohol is filling (or did fill if you've already made the decision to remove alcohol)?

If you are in the very early stages of removing alcohol from your life, make a list of all the reasons you want to do this. I referred to my list many times in my early days of sobriety and it kept me from reaching for a wine on many occasions!

SOBER ACTION STEPS

☐ Consider your own drinking story. When did it start, how did it develop, what brought you to the point you are today? Some women enjoy writing this in the form of a story, letter or blog.

☐ Reflect on the 'magic', 'medicine' and 'misery' stages and decide what stage you are now. How long have you been there?

☐ Be aware of the seven reasons we drink and how many of them are true for you.

☐ Examine how moderation has worked for you in your life: have you ever been a moderate drinker?

☐ Write down all the reasons you want to remove alcohol from your life.

☐ Decide if seeking professional help will benefit you (more on this in Chapter 4).

Commit to 'doing the work'– an incredible, powerful, life-changing exploration and deeply personal journey of self-discovery.

SOBER SISTERS

LEANNE

It was in my mid-40s that I started to question my relationship with alcohol. I distinctly remember my first experience of anxiety. We were flying out to Hawaii for a family holiday and that night my husband and I went out for dinner and polished off a couple of bottles of wine. The next morning as I was getting ready for the airport, I recall shaking with this overwhelming, smothering feeling engulfing my entire body. That was the day I started to really question my relationship with alcohol and I was scared. Scared that I was an alcoholic, scared that I would have to go to AA, scared that I would have to face a life without alcohol being part of it and scared of how I could possibly be happy without ever drinking again – the thought was just not something I wanted to consider.

I spent the next four years exploring sobriety. I didn't think I could live alcohol-free but I realised it was not making me any happier and I was feeling more and more regret whenever I did drink.

So what's happened since I finally, once and for all, quit?

Giving up alcohol has cleared the cobwebs in my brain and I cannot believe what I have achieved. I finally got my scuba diving certification and I have started my Cert IV in Nutrition and enrolled to refresh my Cert IV in Personal Training.

The relationship with my two teenaged children has just grown in leaps and bounds. It was a focus area of mine, to be present and truly engaged and be able to really listen to them. The biggest thing that I was scared of in giving up alcohol was how it would impact the relationship with my husband. He has been my drinking buddy for the past 30 years and a large part of my drinking life. I knew he was also scared about how my decision to give up alcohol would impact us and our life.

I am so happy to say that our relationship is actually better. I am no longer irrational, moody, sad, irritable or snappy. I am now patient and my moods are stable and I am a much happier person, which my husband has openly acknowledged.

My work colleagues all know I don't drink and find it intriguing. We still do lunches and everyone drinks around me but they all respect that I choose not to and treat me exactly the same.

My sleep has improved and I no longer wake at 3 a.m. with my mind racing and unable to get back to sleep. I read books, I journal, I meditate and practise gratitude and positive affirmations, and I see the world with clear eyes and truly see the beauty in my surroundings.

Giving up alcohol has been the best decision I have ever made. I still have fleeting moments when I fantasise about having a drink but they are easily swept aside and I just remind myself how happy and calm I feel now. My only regret is that I didn't do it sooner.

CHAPTER 3
THE SCIENCE BITS

Cravings 101

Picture this. It's 3 a.m. and you wake with a dry mouth, pounding heart and banging head. Slowly your recollections of the night before start to come back to you and you inwardly groan. That 'just popping over to Rachel's for a glass, won't be home late' progressed, like it usually does – one bottle finished, the second bottle opened and oops, also gone. Perhaps even a sneaky fag out the back door and a late-night stumble home. You toss and turn for the next few hours trying desperately to get back to sleep and while you drift in and out of consciousness, deep and restorative sleep eludes you.

By 6.30 a.m. you're up and dressed, making the school lunches, planning the day, and *promising* yourself you won't drink tonight. Nope, definitely not. It's going to be a dry week and you're going to eat well, exercise every day, get to bed early and feel your best. Happy with your newfound discipline and decision, you go about your day. But by 5 p.m., all thoughts of detoxing and kale smoothies and early morning gym sessions are out the window and without truly knowing why, you're cracking open a bottle and the entire cycle starts again. This was my life for years on end. (Yours, too?)

When we drink alcohol, it causes a physiological response in our brain and body that can make practising moderation a myth. And for many of us, we've also created neural pathways that associate the end of the day, unwinding and mitigating stress, with picking up a drink. Those neural pathways are deeply embedded, sometimes for decades. It's not uncommon for me to work with women for whom this has been their hardwired habit for over 40 years. It takes work to rewire those neural pathways, but it *can* be done. We can learn the hacks to work *with* our body to minimise cravings and understand what we need to add *in* when we take alcohol *out*.

But first, what is physically going on in our brain and body when we pick up a drink? What are the biological and behavioural responses that occur?

Knowledge is power when it comes to actually understanding how to physically change our drinking habits and reduce our desire for alcohol.

Your brain on booze

Warning! We're about to get a bit geeky because it's important to understand some of the science behind what happens to our bodies and brains when we drink. This will set us up for all the other chapters that follow. (I'll keep it light, though, and those of you who want to learn more can go to the resources I've added in the back of the book.) Let's start with what neurotransmitters are, how alcohol affects them and why we even need to know this.

Neurotransmitters are chemical messengers that your body can't function without. Their job is to carry chemical signals (messages) from one neuron (nerve cell) to the next.

Our brain is constantly working to maintain a consistent balance of its neurotransmitters at all times, a state that is called homeostasis.

We have well over 100 neurotransmitters in our brains in total but the three we are covering in this chapter are:

1. **Gamma-aminobutyric acid (GABA)**. This helps us feel relaxed and less anxious with a calmer mind, and decreases activity in our nervous system.

2. **Serotonin**. This is responsible for our sense of mental and physical wellbeing encompassing mood, sleep, digestion and levels of happiness.

3. **Dopamine**. This is responsible for feelings of pleasure, satisfaction, reward and motivation.

When we are in homeostasis, our neurotransmitters are balanced and our brain is operating optimally. All is well. We have good mood, memory, physical and emotional wellbeing. When our neurotransmitters are out of balance, this leads to problems with mood, memory, sleep, energy and addictions.

Alcohol disrupts the balance of our neurotransmitters instantly, even after just one glass of wine. If we've been drinking regularly and consistently for years on end (this doesn't have to be in excessive amounts, but just constant and regular alcohol use), this disruption is detrimental to so many factors in both our mental and physical wellbeing and it can take a long time to heal. Never underestimate the impact of even moderate alcohol use on our brain. It's therefore essential that in sobriety, we work to balance our neurotransmitters. Although this can take time, the good news is, it can be done!

Let's consider these three important neurotransmitters and alcohol's impact on each.

While it takes 72 hours for alcohol to physically leave our body, it can take over a year for our neurotransmitters to rebalance after years of consistent drinking.

GABA

GABA is the neurotransmitter that helps us feel calm, relaxed and less anxious. In science terms it is called an 'inhibitory' neurotransmitter because it inhibits brain activities, so reduces overthinking and anxious thoughts. Interestingly, in women, GABA works in correlation with our progesterone hormone. Women who are low in progesterone are often low in GABA, meaning they feel more stressed and anxious. Normally in the second half of our monthly cycle, when progesterone is at its highest, more GABA is released. As we age, however, our progesterone naturally starts declining from our late 30s onwards (as part of the perimenopause stage) which means our GABA levels are impacted, too. If we are deficient in GABA we tend to experience more anxiety, spend more time ruminating and overthinking things, experience increased feelings of stress and overwhelm, and can find it harder to switch off and fall asleep. Are you recognising all this in yourself? I certainly did! I was relieved to actually understand physiologically what was happening in my body as I was ageing and noticing increased feelings of stress, anxious thinking and poor sleep.

It therefore makes sense that if we are deficient in GABA, we are more likely to crave alcohol. GABA is undeniably the neurotransmitter that the majority of the women I work with are highly deficient in (me included). And it helps us understand why this leads to us reaching for alcohol most nights. Let me explain.

Initially alcohol mimics the effects of GABA by inhibiting brain activity. This explains why, when we drink alcohol, we get a warm, fuzzy feeling of relaxation in the first twenty minutes. A study on the impact of alcohol on our neurotransmitters reveals that ethanol, the main component of alcohol, 'acts to depress brain function, very much in the style of an anaesthetic', and in low blood concentration 'releases behaviours that are otherwise inhibited and usually produces feelings of relaxation'.

If we're already deficient in GABA and find it hard to switch off and relax, then we discover that alcohol does this for us, it helps us to understand why we keep going back to it. Because, initially, it works! We wouldn't keep going back to a substance that we know causes so much harm in the long term unless in the moment, it does something for us. Therein lies the problem: we create a neural pathway loop that tells us every time we feel stressed, we should drink alcohol.

However, when we drink alcohol and create that surge of inhibitory neurotransmitters, it causes a disruption to the brain's delicate homeostasis. In order to reclaim that balance, the brain releases alerting chemicals, such as cortisol (a hormone responsible for feelings of stress and anxiety), among others.

As William Porter says in his book *Alcohol Explained:*

Essentially, alcohol provides us with a feeling of relaxation. However, the brain and nervous system reacts to this by releasing stimulants and becoming more sensitive, with the result that when the alcohol wears off we are more anxious and unrelaxed than we were before we took the drink.

So once the alcohol has worn off, we are left with these circulating stimulants that lead us to feel even more stressed and anxious, which in turn makes us more likely to reach for another drink to rid ourselves of the feeling we've created by picking up a drink in the first place. It's madness!

In our efforts to relax ourselves with alcohol, we are causing our brain to release more stimulants, which leads to us feeling more stressed and anxious, the feeling we were trying to escape from in the first place!

Ironically, one of the issues with long-term and consistent alcohol use is that our GABA receptors are reduced and our natural GABA production decreases, which in turn leads to us feeling more anxious or stressed and thus craving more alcohol. And, as we have discussed, our increased consumption of alcohol leads to increased amounts of stimulants being released in the brain. This means that people who drink regularly have an increased level of the stress hormone cortisol circulating in their bodies.

As Andrew Huberman, Associate Professor of Neurobiology at Stanford School of Medicine, explains 'people who drink regularly (even in small amounts, i.e. one per night) experience increases in cortisol release from adrenal glands so feel more stress and more anxiety when not drinking'.

Basically, alcohol is making us *more* stressed and anxious! Ever heard of the term 'hangxiety?' Now you know where it comes from and why we often feel more anxious on the days after drinking. A common quote in the recovery world which sums this madness up perfectly:

Alcohol postpones anxiety and then multiplies it.

Something so many women notice when they remove alcohol is how much their anxiety reduces in a very short time.

Over 80 per cent of the women I work with are GABA deficient. An incredibly useful tool to help you discover if you are deficient in GABA, or any other neurotransmitter, is to complete a self-assessment neurotransmitter questionnaire. (I recommend the Braverman Test, which can be accessed at bravermantest.net.) This is something I do with all my clients so we have factual results to know which neurotransmitters we need to work on replenishing to reduce cravings for alcohol. This information is gold and yet something so few of us know is available to us.

Therefore, one of the most important things we can do when we remove alcohol is work on ways to increase our natural GABA production (more on this later).

SEROTONIN

Serotonin is the chemical in the body responsible for memory, learning and especially for feelings of wellbeing. However, alcohol has a detrimental impact on serotonin levels. The toxic effects of alcohol initially increase serotonin so we can experience a boost of increased happiness and wellbeing, but shortly after, our levels dramatically drop. This can cause or exacerbate feelings of depression.

In the short term, the rise and fall in serotonin leads to us reaching for another drink to simply get back to the baseline of where we were before we had that first drink. And just like GABA, while initially producing feelings of happiness and wellbeing, the long-term use of alcohol often results in a decrease in serotonin, leading to an increase in anxiety and unhappiness.

Something else to consider when it comes to serotonin is that up to 90 per cent of our serotonin is made in the gut. And guess what alcohol does? It disrupts our gut health. It's actually a major cause of leaky gut and plays a key role in killing our good bacteria, while feeding our bad gut bacteria, which means serotonin production is compromised. We also have to remember most alcoholic drinks contain a high amount of sugar, another cause of gut health issues.

Working on replenishing and rebuilding serotonin naturally and improving our gut health is a key factor in reducing our desire to drink and enhancing our sense of wellbeing.

DOPAMINE

I'm saving the best for last! Learning about my dopamine pathways has led to one of the biggest light-bulb moments in my sobriety journey and I am sure this will really resonate with you, too.

Dopamine is the neurotransmitter that plays a role in how we experience pleasure, as well as being a big part of our unique ability to plan, strive, focus and find things interesting.

For many of us alcohol delivers a hefty 'punch' to our brain's dopamine reward centre. When we drink, our brain's reward system is flooded with dopamine. In fact, dopamine levels can increase simply by thinking about having a drink because we have already previously associated alcohol with pleasure. The amount of dopamine that is released depends on the individual – which is why some of us (and many grey area drinkers fall into this category) get a bigger 'punch' from alcohol than others.

Andrew Huberman says you can look around a room of teenagers or young adults drinking and pick the ones who are more likely to go on and develop alcohol use disorder: they are the ones who get more lit up, lively, animated and vivacious with every drink they have. Others may be reaching for water after a couple of drinks or start to feel tired but for those of us that get lit up by alcohol, the signs may have always been there that we would go on to become grey area drinkers. (Can you recognise that lit-up feeling from alcohol? When did you first experience it?)

It's these hefty punches to the reward centre of the brain that can lead to some people developing an addiction to alcohol. Alcohol works in much the same way as other chemicals and behaviours that light up the dopamine pleasure centre: cocaine, methamphetamine, sugar, social media, pornography, gambling. We get a high but what comes up must come down and when we go down, we often land in a trough below where we were to start with, so we crave the substance again to get us out of the trough. Remember, according to Professor David Nutt, alcohol is one of the most addictive substances and this explains why we get lit up, it wears off and then we want more! This is the cycle of addiction. Another compounding issue is that continuous alcohol use down-regulates our dopamine receptors, as it does with GABA, meaning we start to need more and more to get the same high.

However, our brains were not designed to receive the kinds of hard knocks that alcohol provides. They cope much better with more of a 'tickle': a gentle, natural high where we find joy and happiness instead of artificially induced pleasure which always leads to us wanting to go back for more. Think of a tickle as a cuddle with your kids, a great exercise class, laughing with friends, intimate moments with your partner, a great sunrise or sunset. So often we miss the tickles in our bid to get the punches, and part of our work in sobriety is to start noticing the tickles again. These tickles are often called 'glimmers'.

SEARCHING FOR GLIMMERS

Early in therapy, my incredible therapist gave me an exercise to start searching for glimmers every day. It's something I've stuck to all these years and now also practise with my kids, as well as my clients in their early sobriety. Our brain is wired for survival, to always be on the alert for threat and danger, often preparing for the worst, which is known as negativity bias. And one thing I know for sure is that if we look for the negative, we will always find it. But this works the other way too – we can start training our brain to look for and notice the positives in life, no matter how small. These are our glimmers and they are unique to each of us.

To me, glimmers are more authentic and natural than the dopamine punches. An example of a glimmer might be a shared smile with a loved one, experiencing the wonder of an incredible sunset or sunrise at the beach, getting into a bed with clean sheets after a long day at work with a contented sigh, diving into the ocean on a hot day, that warm, fuzzy feeling you get watching your kids laugh and play on the trampoline, a piss-yourself-laughing moment with a close friend at something only the two of you understand, watching your daft dog chase his tail around and around (anyone else got a crazy cocker spaniel like mine?), intimate moments with a loved one or beautiful food shared with your closest friends. These glimmers are experiences and moments that fill us with a warm glow inside. We don't need 'more' because we have exactly what we need in the moment. And when we spend time truly noticing what's always been there, often right under our noses, we begin to feel more positive, more content and more present in our lives. These glimmers may not be as hard-hitting as a bottle of wine or the thrill of ordering a dress you've been coveting for ages, but the impact lasts longer.

The two most common themes I hear when I ask my clients to share their glimmer lists are people and nature. That's where humans find their true, authentic joy – not at the bottom of the bottle or the end of the biscuit packet. They are moments shared with the people we love doing the things we love – simple yet so powerful.

These glimmers may not light us up in quite the palpable way that some of the dopamine punches do, but when we experience authentic happiness, we feel a sense of 'enough', a joy, a sense that everything we need is right with us, and we don't want more. Genuine happiness is a less manic, less in-your-face sensation and a more contented, peaceful, calm feeling.

When we begin to consider how we find joy, it's more helpful to explore the things that provide us with *happiness*, rather than the things that provide us with *pleasure*.

EXERCISE – LOOKING FOR GLIMMERS!

I challenge you to start looking for these little 'free' moments of joy each day. Spoiler alert! You don't need to spend your money on what is being advertised to you! Be on the lookout for the glimmers that give your heart a little lift. The steps below are inspired by Deb Dana's book, *Polyvagal exercises for safety and connection.*

1. Set a goal to look for a certain number of glimmers each day. For me, this number is five.

2. Notice when you feel a fizzle of joy in your tummy, a warm glow of contentment or a surge of upbeat energy.

3. Pause, notice and appreciate the glimmer. You can consider a simple way for you to acknowledge that a glimmer has occurred. You might silently say 'glimmer!' or place a hand on your heart (I do both).

4. Keep track of your glimmers. I write mine in my journal or my phone.

5. Start to notice patterns and then ways in which your glimmers routinely appear so you can be more ready to welcome them. For example, do you always get glimmers on your morning dog walk (a 'good morning' and smile from a stranger, the sun rising over the tops of the trees, swans on the river), sitting at the dinner table with your family, in your yoga studio, or at the beach?

Is your brain on booze like a Christmas tree in Times Square?

When our brain gets lit up several nights a week from alcohol like a bloody Christmas tree in Times Square, we start to anticipate those dopamine punches and look forward to them. We stop noticing the gentler dopamine tickles, the glimmers. Andrew Huberman describes addiction as 'a gentle narrowing of the things from which we find pleasure'. Boom! So true for me. You, too?

I stopped looking forward to or enjoying anything that didn't involve drinking. One of the (many!) incredible benefits of creating a life without booze is that I started noticing the dopamine tickles again. And I realised they were there all along. I'd just forgotten to look for them in my quest for the heavier punches.

LET'S REFLECT

Let's take a moment to reflect on what you might have recognised in yourself from reading this section on neurotransmitters. Later in the chapter I will share strategies for naturally rebalancing our neurotransmitters.

1. How often do you use alcohol to relax and switch off? How often do you feel stressed and anxious the next day? (GABA deficiency)

2. Do you notice a 'high' and quick improvement in mood when you drink, but feel flat and low for the next day or two? (serotonin depletion)

3. How much time do you spend looking forward to and anticipating your next drink? Have you stopped noticing glimmers in your days? (dopamine deficiency)

While you were sleeping

Now you know what alcohol is doing to your brain while you're awake, let's start to look at what is going on while you sleep.

Remember your last alcohol-induced 3 a.m. wake-up, with a dry mouth and racing heart? You toss and turn for hours because, despite feeling really tired, you just cannot return to sleep. Your mind starts wandering, worrying about the day ahead and the fact you're going to be feeling exhausted, and you berate yourself for drinking so much when you promised yourself you wouldn't. All this is caused by the stimulating neurotransmitters your brain has been releasing in response to the alcohol. Once the sedating effects of the booze wears off, you're left with increasing amounts of cortisol racing around your body. And if we drink at night, as most of us do, a few hours later these stimulating neurotransmitters are disrupting our sleep.

Alcohol impacts our sleep in four key ways:

1. When we sleep, we go through several cycles which all include light sleep, rapid eye movement (REM) sleep and deep sleep. All stages of the sleep cycle are essential for promoting brain health, preventing obesity and disease, and promoting healthy ageing and longevity. REM is the cycle associated with dreaming and an incredibly important part of brain health, and deep sleep can promote longevity and the prevention of Alzheimer's and associated dementias. We can average between five to six cycles of sleep a night that include both deep sleep and REM sleep. Yet, scientists have found that when we drink, even just a little, we can bypass many cycles of REM sleep, sometimes reducing them to just one or two full cycles. Lack of REM sleep is linked to obesity, poor learning, low mood, poor heart health and dementia.

2. Alcohol falls into the category known as a sedative, but it's really important to understand that sedation from alcohol is *not* the same as deep sleep. When we are sedated, we switch off brain cells that would ordinarily be firing during the deep sleep stage and which are essential for flushing out toxins and keeping our brain healthy. (This says a lot about why you may experience symptoms similar to a hangover after taking a sleeping tablet.) Neuroscientist and sleep specialist Matthew Walker has a brilliant talk on YouTube explaining this.

3. Alcohol fragments our sleep, which means that although we may fall asleep quickly, it activates our stimulating hormones, which in turn means we wake up a hell of a lot! Fragmented sleep can lead to increased fat mass, increased inflammation, increased insulin resistance, increased leptin levels (meaning we feel more hungry) and increased gut permeability (leaky gut).

4. Alcohol is also known to increase our hot flushes if we are in perimenopause (or even if we're not!) so if you are experiencing night sweats anyway, alcohol will only be exacerbating these.

A process called vasodilation occurs when we drink, which is when the blood vessels in the skin tend to widen. These dilated blood vessels can lead to the skin feeling warmer, which triggers sweat as our body's natural response to help us cool down. Of course, this sweating can occur at any time (the reason why some people get very red in the face when they drink) but as most of us drink in the evening before bed, it's why we can wake up in a pool of sweat a few hours later. For women experiencing hot flushes as a result of hormone fluctuation in menopause, alcohol is only adding fuel to the fire.

If you've ever found yourself saying, 'I'm not hungover, I'm just tired,' now you know why – you simply aren't getting deep, restorative sleep when you drink, even if it is only one or two glasses.

On the nights you can take it or leave it, it's always better to leave it because of the impact on your sleep.

Hormones, menopause and the liver

Before we look at some key strategies to improve our physical health and ways to replenish our neurotransmitters so we can reduce our physical craving for booze, there is one last piece of the puzzle to consider.

Have you ever wondered why, as you've aged, your hangovers have become worse? Or even considered the impact alcohol is having on your hormones, and thus your menstrual cycle? I hadn't.

Drinking in excess is a contributing factor to oestrogen dominance. To explain what that is and why it's important, let me share my own experience. I had been to see my wonderful naturopath, Garth, after suffering from extremely heavy menstrual bleeding and cramps. He conducted some hormone tests and called me a couple of weeks later saying, 'Sarah, your oestrogen is so high it's off the chart. You need to take a break from booze for a while.' I remember feeling confused at first – what on earth did my evening wine have to do with my oestrogen levels – and secondly 'WHATEVER'.

It was December, my favourite month of the year, the only month where it's acceptable to drink in the morning and on Mondays. As if I was going to take a break!

I didn't know then what I know now. Everything we breathe, eat, drink, inject or put on our skin has to be processed and detoxified (cleaned) by our liver, along with the hormones we naturally produce such as oestrogen. Our liver is responsible for over 500 vital functions in our body. It's already working hard, so when we add alcohol to the mix, it has to work overtime. It will always prioritise detoxifying and removing external substances (over anything the body makes itself, like oestrogen) because it considers them more of a threat.

So, if it has to pick, your body will choose to process alcohol over oestrogen. Therefore, when it's constantly ridding your system of alcohol (and caffeine, sugar, processed foods, toxins from skin-care products, make-up and air pollutants), it never gets the chance to move on to the oestrogen and we get a build-up, a state called oestrogen dominance. This is also correlated to our progesterone levels dropping as we age. Symptoms of oestrogen dominance include extremely heavy periods and menstrual cramps, PMS, headaches, mood swings, reduced sex drive, anxiety and depression, and sometimes fibroids.

What's more concerning is that an increase in circulating oestrogen which the liver hasn't had a chance to metabolise is a clear contributing factor to hormone-related cancers. One study shows that drinking alcohol increases circulating oestrogen in the blood by over 20 per cent. According to Avonne Connor, Assistant Professor of Epidemiology at Johns Hopkins University, women who have three alcoholic drinks per week have a 15 per cent higher risk of developing breast cancer. And that risk increases by 10 per cent for every additional drink per day.

It's also really important to mention that when a woman hits the perimenopause years (from late 30s onwards), our liver volume begins to shrink, by 1 to 3 per cent per year. In some cases, by the time we have reached our later years it may have shrunk up to 40 per cent of its original size. (Seriously, most people are astounded at this fact!) When I read this, I had to pause for a moment. There is so much we still don't know about the menopause years and the effect it's having on our body, especially when we throw alcohol into the mix.

This reduction in liver volume means we simply cannot process alcohol in the way men can. In fact, women going through menopause are twice as likely to develop liver disease as men. And this is also considering the fact that women are more vulnerable anyway, as we have already discussed, because we produce fewer of the enzymes that metabolise alcohol (compared to men), before we even throw ageing into the mix. This explains why our hangovers get worse as we age.

I know that some of the facts I have shared here may be confronting and it's never my intention to scaremonger. But it is my intention to share relevant factual information that will allow women to be armed with as much information as possible to live their healthiest, happiest life.

In a world where alcohol is constantly promoted as the path to self-care and reward everywhere we turn, if my little voice in this big world can support women to make informed decisions about their alcohol use, I will keep screaming my message from the rooftops! The good news is that there are so many steps we can take to live our healthiest life without a single alcoholic drink in sight and so much we can do to repair our body after we've made the decision to ditch the booze from our lives. In fact, our incredible liver can begin to repair after just three months of making significant lifestyle changes.

Now is the time to take your own health into your hands and live by the motto: 'I matter and my body comes first.'

Let's add in, not just take out

Now that we've learned about what alcohol is doing to our brain and our bodies, let's get practical with what we can add *in* once we've taken alcohol *out*.

This is the fun part! Not only will this information help reduce physical cravings for alcohol but it will also help us begin to feel our best so we flourish in all areas of our life. The knock-on effect on our relationships, mental wellbeing, self-esteem, work productivity, motivation and energy can never be underestimated. And who doesn't want more of that?

I know it's not sexy or rocket science to talk about the basics but honestly, never take for granted the power of sleeping well, eating well and moving well. These are the three foundational pillars for feeling at your best.

Let's look at each.

SLEEPING

How do you sleep? Really? Do you wake feeling refreshed, energised and ready to take on the day? As you've seen, deep and restorative sleep is essential for our mental and physical wellbeing, which is why I've listed it first here.

We need to rest, replenish and restore our body and brain, and we generally need between seven and eight hours of sleep a night to do this. Why? Because this is how long it takes for the toxins that build up over that day to be removed from our brain, leaving us ready for the next day.

Good sleep plays a major role in reducing our desire for wine. Remember, we are much more likely to self-sabotage when we are tired. For me, tiredness is a huge trigger for craving sugar, not going to the gym, an increase in negative thinking and having a less productive day. Therefore, if I was feeling tired and flat, by the time it rolled round to 5 p.m., the more likely I would have been to hit the 'fuck it' button and reach for wine.

Booze-free sleep will:

- increase energy

- improve concentration

- replenish neurotransmitters (especially dopamine)

- enable better memory and greater capacity to learn

- reduce stress levels

- support weight loss

- increase life expectancy.

Remember that when we are making big changes in our lives and doing something differently (in this case, not drinking), it takes up lots of energy in our brain. Until this becomes the new normal, our brain is having to work hard to resist the pattern of drinking. This can make us feel extra tired, and it's not uncommon in the early days of sobriety to find you are sleeping longer than usual but still feeling tired the next day.

So many people are surprised by this – they think that they should bounce out of bed immediately after removing alcohol – but it doesn't work like that. If we've been drinking consistently for years, we can't expect our body to bounce back in a weekend. It takes time and we have to be patient and give our healing body what it needs – in this case more sleep and rest.

Some easy actionable tips for better sleep include:

- **An hour before your ideal bedtime eliminate screen time and turn down the lights in your home**. This increases your production of our natural sleep hormone, melatonin. Make sure your bedroom is dark, cool and free of screens – sleeping with a phone by our bed makes our brain more hypervigilant and reduces the quality of our sleep.

- **Use calming scents to relax**. Our sense of smell sends a rapid message to the brain to relax. I love vetiver essential oil and most nights I will have this burning in my diffuser, added to a bath or mixed with my body lotion and rubbed into my skin. It works wonders for deep sleep.

- **Set up your day for a great sleep**. Getting natural sunlight on your retinas early in the morning is the best way to support falling asleep easily. This is because the sunlight causes a sharp rise in cortisol, our 'get up and go' hormone. We want this to be high in the morning and low at night. When cortisol is high first thing, it means its opposing hormone, melatonin (our sleep hormone), is low in the morning and then rises at night, when we want it to. Aim for 'ten before ten' (ten minutes of sunlight before 10 a.m.). Having your morning cup of tea in the garden (without sunglasses!) is a great hack for this or adding in a morning stroll or exercise outside. Reducing caffeine and sugar consumption, especially after lunch, can also have a huge impact on our sleep, as they both cause us to release cortisol. Eating no less than two hours before bed helps as well. Try to avoid exercise in the evening as this can also raise your cortisol levels. Fun fact – pistachios are one of the foods with a high amount of melatonin! Eating a handful after dinner is a great idea.

THE PHYSICAL IMPACT
OF SOBRIETY

'I can't believe how much my
memory and recall has improved!'

NAOMI

'My nails and hair are growing much
more quickly, my teeth are so much
whiter (red wine drinker), and I've
lost weight without trying.'

ELLIE

'The significant change in
menopause symptoms.'

ALISON

LET'S REFLECT

1. How often do you fall asleep easily and stay asleep through the night?

2. How often do you wake feeling refreshed, energised and well rested?

3. How often do you wake at the same time each day without needing an alarm?

If answering these questions is creating some red flags for you in terms of your sleep, consider the tips I've mentioned on page 65 and decide which you will prioritise to begin with. Never underestimate the importance of a good sleep for improving your mood and wellbeing, and reducing your desire for alcohol.

EATING

Many of us are living on a blood sugar roller-coaster, every single day, and as well as impacting our mood and energy, it's not helping with our booze cravings either.

Any food containing high amounts of sugar and starch (which includes most processed foods, sweet treats and soft drinks) causes an increase in blood sugar, which can then lead to a big drop and initiate cravings to raise our levels again. We can be on this roller-coaster all day without even realising it. Let's consider for a moment an average Western-style breakfast. It usually consists of some kind of cereal (containing on average nine teaspoons of sugar), yoghurt (if flavoured, on average five teaspoons of sugar), a milky coffee (three teaspoons) and/or a glass of juice (five teaspoons). Eating this style of breakfast can cause a huge blood sugar spike as it contains up to 22 teaspoons of sugar. The World Health Organization advises we have no more than six teaspoons in a day for the best health benefits – and we've just had almost four times that amount at breakfast!

While this sugar hit gives us a surge of energy (hooray!), a couple of hours later we crash and burn (boo!), so our brain sends out a message to eat more sugar/starch to get out of the crash. We then reach for a coffee and cake, a bagel, a muffin or any other sweet treat which leads to another high. And then this is followed by another low. And so it continues all day and into the evening.

BLOOD SUGAR

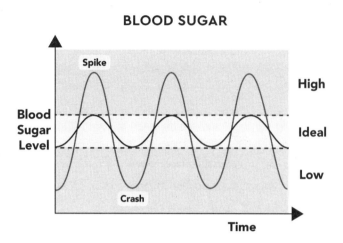

By the time it gets to 5 p.m. we have been on this glucose roller-coaster of spikes and crashes for hours, and guess what our brain is going to start screaming for to get us out of that trough? Yep, our nightly sugary, alcoholic drink. Sometimes I bypassed dinner altogether and simply drank my evening meal.

Some facts for you (and remember most government health policies' daily recommended allowance of sugar is a maximum of twelve teaspoons:

- a schooner or pint of beer/ale = up to 9 teaspoons of sugar
- a large glass of medium white wine = up to 3 teaspoons of sugar
- a pint of cider = up to 10 teaspoons of sugar
- a gin and tonic = up to 4 teaspoons of sugar
- an espresso martini = up to 5 teaspoons of sugar.

Being on this constant sugar roller-coaster only exacerbates our alcohol cravings, which is why being strategic with *what* and *when* we eat can help reduce these cravings. Maintaining balanced blood-sugar levels through the day is key to reducing cravings. One hack I love is to have a nutritious snack at around 3 p.m. to combat the 5 p.m. cravings – an apple with some nut butter, chicken slices with avocado on a rice cracker or a couple of boiled eggs and some almonds. Works a treat for me and so many of my clients! Keeping your blood sugar balanced will also help to improve your mood, energy, sleep and cognition.

There is simply so much power in understanding *how* to eat in order to reduce our desire for alcohol. And none of this is about dieting or calories: it's all about improving mental wellbeing, sleep and energy. Here are some suggestions to get you started:

- **Eat regular amounts of protein and leafy greens**. The amino acids in protein support our neurotransmitter production (especially of serotonin and dopamine), as well as help balance blood sugars and reduce blood sugar spikes. Eating more nuts, seeds, eggs, turkey, chicken, beef, cheese and plain yoghurt throughout the day reduces cravings for sugary foods and alcohol. Add in lots of dark green veggies (broccoli is your liver's best friend), and ensure you are drinking 2 litres of water a day to help carry essential nutrients to your cells.

- **Try fermented foods to improve your gut health and support your production of GABA, serotonin and dopamine**. I eat sauerkraut, miso, kefir or kimchi every day. Feeding our good gut bacteria and starving our bad gut bacteria (by removing alcohol and as much sugar and processed food as we can) really makes a difference. We also do this by ensuring we get a wide variety of different fruit, veg, nuts, seeds, herbs, spices and legumes each week.

- **Consult a naturopath or doctor to run blood tests and see if you need supplements**. Magnesium is the mineral we burn through the most when we are stressed. Many of us are deficient in magnesium – I personally love soaking in an Epsom salts bath or taking a night-time magnesium supplement before bed. Other vitamins that can be helpful in improving our wellbeing include B-vitamins, zinc, L-theanine (which supports GABA production), and vitamin D – especially in winter. (Vitamin D supports our neurotransmitter production, particularly serotonin.)

Dr Helena Popovic says that drinking three alcoholic drinks a night depletes our levels of B1, which can put us at risk of a specific type of dementia called Wernicke-Korsakoff Syndrome (WKS), another good reason to supplement with vitamin B. Certain supplements can really boost your liver function, too. I recommend speaking to a qualified naturopath or functional medicine nutritionist to identify exactly what to add in for *you*. Don't just run to the chemist and buy everything as it can be damaging to take something you don't actually need.

Finally, just note that if you have removed alcohol it is really, really normal to suddenly crave sugar like you never have before! I have clients who've never had a sweet tooth hiding in the pantry mainlining chocolate biscuits and being unable to stop. These cravings for sugar do subside once your body adjusts. Make sure you're eating really well during this time with a great variety of leafy greens, good-quality fats and regular amounts of protein. Add a small, sugary snack if you need to but don't reach for these sugary items in place of nutritious food.

Learning how to get off the glucose roller-coaster is a huge step forward to managing alcohol cravings.

LET'S REFLECT

1. How regularly are you feeling hungry throughout the day and craving sugary and starchy foods, but then find you are hungry again a couple of hours after eating?

2. Reflect on the last week or so. How many times did you feel tired and lethargic after lunch and want to crawl under your desk for a nap?

3. How often do you experience bloating and/or digestive issues?

4. How many times a week do you crave alcohol by 5 p.m. to give you a 'lift' to get through the evening?

MOVING

In one of my recent alcohol-free challenges, I interviewed eight inspiring guest experts about their journey to sobriety. In every interview, when I asked the question: 'What are your tips for sobriety?', every single interviewee replied: 'Exercise'.

The simplest reason is that exercise makes us feel good! It leads to a surge in dopamine, so if we're getting those dopamine tickles from exercise we are less likely to crave the bottle. Exercise also increases our baseline of dopamine in the body, which is important so we don't fall into dopamine deficiency when we remove alcohol.

Our body was designed to move and yet so many of us live such sedentary lives. We drive to work, sit at a desk all day, drive home, sit for dinner and then sit on the sofa. Finding ways to change this up and get regular movement through the day is so important for both our physical and mental health. In fact, exercise has been shown to treat 26 chronic diseases!

After I quit drinking, I signed up for a half marathon to see what my body could actually do when I wasn't training with alcohol in my system, and I took six minutes off my previous half marathon time! It also gave me a goal, a focus, and something to keep committed to. It also helped me to explain why I wasn't drinking at social events. Not many people argued when I said I had to get up at 5 a.m. to run 18 kilometres, and this really helped calm some of my initial social anxiety. Now, I'm not saying you have to do the same and sign up to the next half marathon, but it really helps to add in some kind of movement every day if you can.

Remember:

- **Take regular movement breaks through the day to get quick dopamine hits**. If we are getting these small regular hits through the day we won't have such a craving for the alcohol hit at night. We also know that regular bursts of movement through the day increases our cognitive function and sense of wellbeing. This can include stretching, running on the spot for 30 seconds, or taking a quick walk around the house or outside.

- **Cardio**! It increases endorphins, which increase feelings of euphoria as well as supporting serotonin and dopamine production. So many of my clients find that taking up running or cycling really supports them on their sobriety journey and diminishes their desire to drink because they are getting that high naturally.

- **Have fun exploring your exercise of choice**. We don't have to all turn into F45 junkies! For some it's hiking, others it's Zumba or peloton. Brisk walking, jogging, dancing, cycling or HIIT classes all increase our feel-good hormone, serotonin, which again means we don't crave the alcohol. A double whammy if we're doing it outside as sunlight also increases serotonin.

LET'S REFLECT

1. What's your current exercise routine?

2. What would you like to try to add into your daily routine that moves your body?

3. What kind of movement do you know makes you feel good?

Happy (natural) neuro-boosting hacks

Finally, before we move on to the next chapter, here are three of my favourite happy hacks that I always try to include when I'm planning my day to support neurotransmitter balance and production.

BOOST YOUR GABA BY MOOD OR FOOD TO REDUCE ANXIETY AND FEEL CALMER

A Boston University School of Medicine study found that just one 60-minute meditation session increased GABA by 27 per cent. Other activities that support GABA production include anything that gives us a calm sense of 'flow' (being lost in the moment) such as reading, cooking, gardening, walking, knitting or doing the crossword. There are also certain foods that aid GABA production including bananas, almonds, broccoli, beef liver, oats and fish (halibut). Finally, never underestimate the power of music for improving mood – it boosts dopamine, serotonin and oxytocin! Create playlists that make you feel happy and uplifted through the day or soothe you at the end of the day.

HAVE FUN IN THE SUN AND EAT WELL FOR SEROTONIN

Natural sunlight and aerobic exercise such as brisk walking, dancing, cycling and running have all been shown to increase serotonin. Make sure you eat plenty of foods that contain tryptophan – an amino acid from protein that converts into serotonin in the body. Tryptophan-rich foods include chicken, turkey, eggs, fish, cheese, pumpkin and sesame seeds. Prioritise your gut health and check your vitamin D levels. As I've mentioned, low vitamin D can impact our serotonin production and some of us may need a supplement, especially in winter months when we have less sunlight.

PRIORITISE DAILY DOPAMINE HITS

Increasing our baseline of dopamine is essential to reduce our cravings for alcohol and there are so many ways we can do this! Dopamine is made from tyrosine or phenylalanine, which is found in protein-rich foods like beef, pork, fish, chicken, seeds and cheese. Exercising regularly increases dopamine (and interestingly, prolonged sitting lowers dopamine!) Make new habits around physical activity a daily priority. Sleep is also important – even one poor night's sleep down-regulates our dopamine receptors. Adding in some practices which encourage deep relaxation, such as NSDR (non-sleep deep rest) or a form of meditation called yoga nidra, is the next best thing for dopamine. Listening to music and picking hobbies that challenge and interest us also help with dopamine production. And for enhanced dopamine throughout your day, start with a cold shower or ice bath – this can increase our dopamine for up to six hours!

COMPLETE THIS SENTENCE

Out of the three pillars of nutrition, sleep and movement, I am going to prioritise improving my _____. This is important to me because _____ and the first step I am taking towards working on this is to _____. I will do this by the following date: _____.

Don't underestimate the impact that good nutrition, regular movement and deep, restorative sleep can have on improving mental wellbeing and reducing physical stress (which we'll look at next).

SOBER ACTION STEPS

☐ Understand the impact that the three pillars of nutrition, sleep and movement have on our cravings for alcohol.

☐ Reflect on your current sleep, nutrition and movement habits – what's going well and where is there room for improvement?

☐ Pick one pillar to begin with. Don't try and change too much at once. If you realise you want to work on all of them, there's no rush! Start with small steps. Once you've worked on the first pillar for a couple of weeks and feel it's on track, move on to the next.

NICOLA

My whole mindset changed since giving up alcohol in my mid-40s. A concept that I love is seeking out 'dopamine tickles' rather than the big dopamine hit you get when you down a large glass of vino. I find these dopamine tickles in the simple things in life – laughing with my kids and friends, playing with pets, music, dancing, a beautiful sunny day, the ocean, coffee and chocolate.

I have discovered so many benefits from not drinking alcohol. There are the obvious physical benefits, including brighter eyes, clearer skin and glossier hair. People often remark how much younger and well I look. I have never really struggled with my weight; however, my waist was widening due to middle-age spread. Giving up alcohol has given me a slim waist again and any excess kilos have disappeared. Forget the fad diets – giving up wine is the easiest way to lose weight! My sleep has much improved, and I no longer wake up around 3 a.m. with a racing mind worrying about everything and anything.

The mental benefits of an alcohol-free life are amazing. I am much calmer and more even-tempered. My relationships with my husband and children have improved considerably. I feel much more joyful, optimistic and confident. I am much more present in everything I do. My life is anything but boring. I also feel freer and am enjoying my life much more. From a social perspective, I am no longer a liability and instead am great fun to be around.

I am not judgemental of other people drinking. I am a big believer in freedom of choice. What I do notice is that most people just relax and enjoy themselves and don't get hideously drunk. I do feel shame with regards to how I used to behave, but I am making the change and that is in the past, so I don't dwell on this thought for long. Another benefit is that I can drive home. No more arguments with my husband about whose turn it is to drive! It really does make everything much simpler than before. I thought I gained freedom from drinking; when, in fact, you gain far greater freedom with sobriety.

I have replaced alcohol with so many beneficial activities including yoga and meditation. I used to have a glass of wine to signal that the workday had ended but now practice Yoga nidra instead. I still do a fair amount of aerobic exercise but now focus on nurturing my body rather than punishing it. I incorporate exercise in my daily routine and mix it up with more intense training some days and more gentle exercises on other days. This kindness to myself, rather than punishment, has come about because of removing alcohol.

To be honest, I did love drinking but it simply does not enhance my life in any way, so I have decided not to go down that path anymore. Always a rebel at heart, I believe that giving up alcohol is breaking the mould, going against Western society norms and, in contrast to the ladette culture of the 1990s, is spearheading the new cool for the 2020s!

CHAPTER 4
FEELING JUMPY?

How to soothe stress

How often do you end the day uttering the words, 'I'm so stressed' with your heart racing, shoulders tensed and tummy in knots? And how often do you catch yourself saying these words as you open the fridge and pour a wine, seeking temporary oblivion from the overwhelming events of the day that's been?

If you're anything like I was, this has likely been your go-to solution to stress for years. I lived on autopilot with the slightest of incidents sending me straight to the fridge as my solution to how I was feeling. (I mean, show me a middle-aged woman who isn't stressed about something? I don't know any … do you?)

**Alcohol has become a free-and-easy solution to stress,
yet it's only adding to the problem!**

The women I work with all say the most common reasons for drinking are stress and feelings of overwhelm. We have a generation of women who constantly feel so stressed and overwhelmed that they're living close to extreme burnout and whose only tool each evening is seeking solace in a glass of wine (or three). And as we've discussed, Big Alcohol's marketing has only amplified our justification that we *need* and *deserve* alcohol to unwind after a hard day.

Why does stress lead us to drink?

Alcohol, as we know, is a depressant, which means it works on the inhibitory neurotransmitters in the brain (remember our science lesson in Chapter 3?). It leads to us feeling calmer and more relaxed. And if we're living in a state of constantly feeling stressed and overwhelmed, as well as being in the stage of our lives where our progesterone hormone is dropping and we are more deficient in GABA, it makes sense we are going to be drawn to something that calms us down. We're not stupid, we wouldn't keep going back to it time and time again if it didn't actually do what we wanted it to. But while reaching for a drink seems like a good short-term solution, in the long term we're making it a hell of a lot worse. And as we've already discussed, if we want to successfully change or end our relationship with alcohol, we need to look at the root cause of the trigger (in this case, stress) and deal with *that* first so our need for alcohol simply isn't as strong.

We also have to remember that we currently have a global epidemic of stress. It's become so normal that I believe we've almost lost sight of what it feels like to *not* feel stress. The World Health Organization calls it the greatest health risk of the 21st century, and it is linked to many more health conditions and diseases than we first thought.

More and more research is revealing the impact stress plays in diseases such as type 2 diabetes, heart disease, stroke, obesity, anxiety and depression.

And then there's menopause. Increased stress also plays a major role in how severely we experience menopause symptoms, and menopause also *causes* us to experience stress because of the hormone changes that are occurring. It's another vicious cycle. When I interviewed Dr Wendy Sweet (PhD), a leading menopause expert, she said:

Numerous women find that they feel more stressed and anxious as they navigate menopause. There's a reason for this – as the reproductive hormones are declining, the body is ageing, and this includes the ageing of the adrenal glands, where stress hormones are produced.

As such, the ageing adrenals produce more of the chronic stress hormone called cortisol, which in turn, contributes to imbalances in the main hormonal axis, called the hypothalamus-pituitary-adrenal axis (HPA axis).

When this axis gets out of balance during the menopause transition, and because the adrenals are ageing, cortisol levels may remain higher than normal. As such, this can be problematic for sleep, anxiety, brain fog and inflammation.

Over time, chronic stress (including physical stress from too much exercise) can lead to both mental and physical health problems as women age, especially cardiovascular disease. Hence, understanding the lifestyle strategies that reduce stress is an important target for midlife women.

It's just another challenge women face as we age – as we enter our perimenopause years (which is often from our late 30s when we are juggling more than ever in terms of work, kids and ageing parents), physical changes in our body are only adding to the stress. This is another reason why drinking during perimenopause years isn't a good idea.

As we've already discussed, when we drink we actually release stimulating hormones including the stress hormone cortisol, which means when the alcohol wears off, we are left with more cortisol in our body and a greater feeling of stress than before we even picked up a drink.

> **We need to explore what is happening in our body when we experience feelings of stress so we can create healthier solutions.**

It's an ongoing vicious cycle: we drink as a solution to our stress, but the alcohol is making us feel more stressed and anxious, including the following day, so we drink again. And while we should never blame ourselves for using alcohol in the way we have in the past or still do, it is important we begin to work on healthier strategies for reducing stress. In this chapter we are going to explore two types of stress: the stressors that show up in our everyday lives and the accumulated, stored stress in our bodies that may have been with us for years.

Identifying everyday stress

Each day you experience situations, thoughts and events that cause you some degree of stress: sleeping through the alarm and having a mad scramble to get everything done in the morning, turning on the news and seeing there has been a horrendous earthquake with many lives lost, realising you don't have enough bread to make school lunches, skipping breakfast and only having caffeine to fuel your body, doing extensive cardio workouts, missing the train to work and then being late for an important meeting, checking work emails before you go to bed and seeing an email that you can't stop thinking about and then not sleeping well. The list is endless.

These everyday examples happen time and time again. While some are unavoidable, we can also make choices every day that move us towards (or away from) this stressed state, and which we can experience in a completely different way when we have a more regulated and flexible nervous system (which we'll get into in a moment).

Of course, stress is always going to be a part of our lives. We can't completely avoid it in our modern world. However, we can decide how we respond to it and we can make small swaps and changes that impact the stressors we expose ourselves to.

> We can't find freedom from booze if we don't have any
> other tools for managing stress in our modern world,
> because stress isn't going anywhere soon.

As shown in the image opposite, there are things in life we can't control, such as other people's actions, external factors like the weather, or what people think of us or what may happen in the future. Yet we *can* control how well we look after ourselves, what we eat, what time we go to bed,

OUT OF MY CONTROL

The past

The future

The actions
of others

The opinions
of others

IN MY CONTROL

My boundaries

My thoughts and actions

The goals I set

How I speak to myself

What I give my
energy to

How I handle
challenges

What happens
around me

What other
people think
of me

The outcome
of my efforts

How others take
care of themselves

what information we choose to consume, and make sure we have the tools in place to support and protect our emotional wellbeing, our time and our energy so we are in a strong position to better respond to those external factors.

Consider for a moment what your current coping strategies are when you are experiencing times of stress.

- *When stressful situations happen, my go-to response is* _____ *which leaves me feeling* _____.

- *If I take steps to prioritise what is in my control to create a positive influence on my responses, thoughts and actions, I will feel* _____. *This is important to me because* _____.

LET'S REFLECT

Take a moment to consider what the everyday stressors are in your life.

Is it too much caffeine? Too much social media? Too much to do in a short space of time in the morning? Not exercising and never taking time for yourself? Too much cardio? A poor diet? A boss who has no respect for your work–life balance? Kids who leave mess everywhere and don't help clear it up? The evening routine of getting dinner, kids' homework, dogs that need walking?

Make a list of the top six (yes, only six!) stressors for you. We will come back to this shortly.

1. _____

2. _____

3. _____

4. _____

5. _____

6. _____

What happens when we begin to experience stress?

It's in our nervous system that our stress response takes place. We have two branches of the nervous system: sympathetic and parasympathetic. The sympathetic branch is the one that becomes activated when we experience a stressor and the parasympathetic branch is where we remain when we are not experiencing stress. This branch is also known as 'rest and digest'. Having some understanding of our nervous system and stress response not only helps us understand why we might be turning to alcohol so often but also creates awareness around activities and exercises that reduce our feelings of stress.

The stress response comes from a part of our brain called the amygdala. It sends a message to our organs and muscles that we are under threat and in danger and we must prepare for imminent attack! It's a primal response that has supported human evolution for centuries. Our incredible body treats every feeling of stress as if our life is in danger and we're about to come face to face with a grizzly bear in the woods (like our ancestors might have) because that is the purpose of the stress response – to prepare our body for potential danger and ensure our survival. The problem is, our body hasn't caught up with the modern world and doesn't understand we are engaging our stress response as a reaction to the 400 unread emails in our inbox, kids fighting over whose turn it is to walk the dog, or a to-do list that's never-ending. Not a grizzly bear in sight!

Once the amygdala has sent out this 'imminent danger' message, a chain of physical responses commences. Our heart rate increases, our breathing quickens, our muscles tighten and engage, our blood pressure rises, our jaw clenches, our digestion pauses, blood leaves the internal organs to head straight to our outer extremities and we are prepped and primed, ready for 'fight or flight' (meaning that we are ready to either 'battle' our predator or 'run away from' our predator).

But as I said, nearly every time we engage this response, our lives are not actually in danger. It's just that our body doesn't have an alternative response. It *perceives* any stress response to mean our lives are in danger. And this is where the problem lies.

While our ancestors' lives may have been at risk and they used these physical responses as if their lives depended on it (because they did), that's not true for us in our modern world. We don't need to use the excess adrenalin that our adrenals release, we don't need our digestion to pause or our jaw to clench in response to the stress of a missed train or too much caffeine. But our body simply doesn't have another way to respond to stress. And another fact to consider is that, for the most part, our ancestors were perhaps facing this threat once a week at most and entering the stress state for perhaps twenty minutes – just enough time to get them out of the danger zone (and escape that grizzly bear). As we saw earlier, this stress response state is called the sympathetic state and our bodies are built to cope with it for only about twenty minutes before they return to 'normal' (our parasympathetic state).

The issue for us today is that these stressors are coming at us thick and fast all day long, and some of us are living in this stress response state for hours or days on end. Sometimes even years. We get stuck in this state and can't get back to our calmer, baseline state. I was stuck there for years, decades really, but I just had no idea. The feeling of adrenaline flooding my body, my jaw clenching and my tummy tightening simply became my new normal. I find this also to be the case for many women I work with.

When we end up staying stuck in the sympathetic state for too long, we enter what Dr Wayne Todd, a leading authority and practitioner on the sympathetic nervous system, calls 'sympathetic dominance' (and others call hyper arousal), which plays havoc with our mental and physical health.

Sympathetic dominance is when we are spending more time in the sympathetic state than the parasympathetic, 'rest or digest' state, demonstrating symptoms such as tight jaw, grinding teeth, hyperventilation, digestive issues, poor immune system (experiencing frequent colds and flu) and sleep issues.

Have a look through this list of signs of sympathetic dominance from Dr Wayne Todd. How many you can tick off?

- ☐ regular headaches or migraines
- ☐ sensitivity to light or noise
- ☐ tightness in your neck and shoulders (oh yes!)
- ☐ feeling wound up or wired and finding it hard to calm down
- ☐ often feeling cold
- ☐ craving sugar or salt
- ☐ high blood pressure
- ☐ digestive issues (IBS, bloating, constipation, diverticulitis)
- ☐ finding it difficult to lose weight

- [ ] finding yourself tired or low on energy

- [ ] suffering from adrenal exhaustion or fatigue

- [ ] sleeping lightly, with vivid dreams and often waking through the night

- [ ] hormonal issues including oestrogen dominance (heavy periods, clotting, extreme PMS)

- [ ] polycystic ovarian syndrome

- [ ] gall bladder problems or thyroid imbalances

- [ ] hair loss

- [ ] water retention

- [ ] feelings of low mood, depression or anxiety

- [ ] irritability

The first time I read this list I could tick off most of them. What about you? I was particularly interested in the impact of sympathetic dominance on my digestive issues and menstrual cycle.

As someone who ended up in hospital with cameras down my throat and up the other end (cringe) to diagnose acute diverticulitis and bowel polyps, as well as having ongoing issues with polycystic ovarian syndrome, irregular periods, problems conceiving and adrenal fatigue, I was absolutely fascinated at how these conditions were related to my nervous system and my constant feelings of stress. You see, when your body has you prepped to always be ready to fight off that fictional grizzly bear, it puts a hold on digestion, reproduction and anything else not immediately vital to fighting or running. (This makes sense – why would our body think we were ready to make babies or digest food when there's a bear to escape from!) In my case, it took over two years to conceive, and I had ongoing digestive problems and severe oestrogen dominance. I kept being told to 'relax more' and 'not be so stressed' but I was never actually offered any tools on *how* to do this. Over time, I've read, researched, learnt and listened to so much information on this topic that I've built a robust and comprehensive stress-busting toolkit that I will be sharing with you soon!

The beauty of calm

When we are in the parasympathetic state, our internal organs are functioning well. In this state our saliva production is stimulated which aids food digestion, our heart rate slows, our breathing deepens and lengthens, our sexual organs work optimally meaning we have a healthy sex drive, our periods are regular, our bowel movements are classed as healthy and our thyroid and gall bladder operate optimally. We sleep well, feel calm and relaxed and if something does cause a little stress, after an initial burst of fight or flight energy we quickly return to parasympathetic.

This is our body's default operating state, our 'thrive' state that we are designed to be in most of the time, but this simply isn't the case for many of us. More and more of us are living with the fight or flight state as our 'normal.' And it's why we are turning to alcohol so much – when we are constantly in a hyper alert, tense and agitated state, our bodies are crying out for something that relaxes us, and that's what alcohol does in the moment.

The fact that it goes on to make us feel more stressed is irrelevant to our brain at this point – our neural wiring is well established by now and we only remember alcohol soothes us in the moment. It's why we reach for a drink on autopilot when we feel this way. Our brain wants to keep us safe and it's not thinking about the hangover the next morning – only the fact it will relax us right now. Once we have used alcohol as a response to stress (and it worked in the moment) the neural pathway is created and that's what our brain will trigger us to do every time we feel stressed. It's why so many of us find our innocent glass of wine 'to take the edge off' has increased so much over time – the more stress we have, the more we reach for a drink as a solution, and the more regularly we drink, the more tolerance we build to the alcohol, so we need more and more to get the relaxed state we crave. It's a common theme among the women I work with and a common theme for grey area drinkers.

Grey area drinkers are often living life stuck in the flight or fight response state, using alcohol as the solution.

Freeze!

When we have been living in fight or flight for too long, our body recognises that we can't stay in this hypervigilant state indefinitely due to the impact it has on our health (and all those symptoms of sympathetic dominance we've looked at). As a survival mechanism, our body will sometimes go into a 'freeze' state. (I say sometimes because it always amazes me how some people have the capacity to live in that chronic fight or flight state for really prolonged periods – this was certainly the case for me).

In the freeze state, we become inactive. The freeze response can show up as illness, forcing us to rest or withdraw from our lives, society, our friends. It can show up as indecision and inability to act (procrastination). It can show up as chronic exhaustion. It can show up as depression. It can also show up as absolute burnout where we can't even lift our head off the pillow.

For me, the freeze state would show up after months living in that heightened state of fight or flight, burning the candle at both ends with little time for myself. Then bang! Out of nowhere I would be struck down with an unexplained virus that would have me in bed for days on end with no energy, and sleeping twelve to fourteen hours at a time. Despite numerous doctor's visits, there was never a known cause for these mysterious viruses. Of course there wasn't! I was suffering extreme burnout from living for so long in the fight or flight response and my body was finding any way it could to make me stop.

What I now know is that it was my body's way of shutting down when I had been in fight or flight for too long. It wasn't sustainable for me to continue operating in this state of hypervigilance, combined with the amount I was drinking, plus getting poor sleep, having a crap diet and working long hours. Therefore, my body was simply finding a way to put me out of action and force me to rest and recover. I spent years oscillating between living in a state of stress and then being hit with viruses. My poor body.

Never underestimate the power of the human body and the impact our nervous system dysregulation has on our health. Or how it's driving our drinking habits.

What ongoing or mysterious illnesses have shown up for you over the years? Do you recognise being in cycles of fight or flight for long periods of time, followed by the freeze state?

Understanding nervous system flexibility

Understanding how your nervous system works, being able to identify when you are entering a 'stressed' state and having a robust toolkit of resources to both prevent the build-up of stress and to turn to when it occurs is key to no longer *needing* to reach for booze come the end of each stressful, busy day.

I am yet to work with a client whose nervous system is not dysregulated in some way, where they've become 'stuck' in the stress response. This is why so many of the resources I share in my coaching towards sobriety are those which focus on nervous system regulation. I don't believe we can truly remove our desire for alcohol if we don't work to create a more flexible nervous system to enable us to move out of sympathetic dominance.

What do I mean by a 'flexible' nervous system? When our nervous system is regulated, we manage stress well and can quickly return to our rest and digest parasympathetic state once a stressful situation has passed. A flexible nervous system can be one that can access the energy of the stress response when it needs to (and to be clear, we use this response all the time, it's not 'bad' and is super helpful in certain scenarios – if you had to run from someone trying to mug you, if a car mounted the footpath and came towards you and you jumped out of the way, if you needed a surge of energy ready for a presentation at work), but can then drop back down to baseline (the parasympathetic state) soon after. We can also drop down into freeze if we need to (for example it could save our life if we cut ourselves badly by slowing down our heart rate to stop us bleeding out). Nervous system regulation means we move fluidly between states but always return to parasympathetic 'baseline' state by default. Nervous system dysregulation is when we get stuck and can't drop back down to baseline. Some of us have been stuck here for so long, we don't even know what baseline feels like.

Let's look at the table opposite to help you to consider the three different states of our nervous system. Consider how much time you spend in each state on an average day. Is the thrive state your dominant state? A healthy and flexible nervous system is one mostly sitting in the parasympathetic state.

NERVOUS SYSTEM STATE	HOW IT FEELS IN THE BODY	HOW IT FEELS IN THE MIND
Parasympathetic – rest and digest, 'thrive' state: our baseline	Relaxed, peaceful, light, free, healthy function of all organs in the body, optimal health	Joyful, socially engaged, positive, emotionally regulated, connected both to self and others
Sympathetic arousal – fight or flight state	Racing heart, tense muscles, dry mouth, tight tummy, sweaty hands, shoulders hunched, alert, vigilant, sensitive to light and sound	Anxious thoughts, panicked, overwhelmed, fearful, irrational responses, negative thinking, pressure, flooded with emotions
Freeze state	Slow, lethargic, numb, empty, flaccid, exhausted, withdrawn, shut down, ill	Disengaged, withdrawn, disinterested in everything, lack of confidence, don't want to speak

Ending the stress cycle

Let's go back to our primeval ancestor coming face to face with the grizzly bear. All the physical symptoms of entering fight or flight kick in: heart rate increases, breathing quickens, muscles tense, jaw clenches and cortisol and adrenaline course through the body, allowing them to run faster or fight harder to save their own life. And then let's consider you sitting at your desk feeling utterly overwhelmed with your inbox and to-do list, having a strong coffee and experiencing all those same symptoms. What's the main difference?

The difference is that our ancestor *uses* the physical tools that their sympathetic response has offered them in order to fight against the danger. They fight or flee and use that excess energy that their body has offered them. They *end* the stress cycle by using the energy. When you and I have the same response sitting at our desk or in a traffic jam on the freeway, we don't actually use the increased adrenaline and cortisol so it stays stuck in our bodies, coursing round and round for hours. I will be sharing with you later some simple strategies to ensure you can start ending your own stress cycles.

> An important part of the process of the stress cycle is that we actually use and discharge the adrenaline we have created so our body knows the cycle is complete and we can return to the parasympathetic state.

LET'S REFLECT

One of the simplest ways to consider if we are coping well with our everyday stress or whether we have become stuck in a response that leads to nervous system dysregulation is to reflect on how we respond to small stressors through the day.

☐ Do you overreact when the kids knock over a coffee cup?

☐ Do you feel constantly alert and anxious?

☐ If you find yourself with a spare couple of hours at the weekend with no one around, can you easily relax, read a book or watch a movie, or do you find you always have to be 'doing' something?

☐ How many times a day is your response greater than the situation requires?

It's also important we consider if we have stored stress stemming from the past, which may mean we have been living with nervous system dysregulation for much of our lives.

Exploring our stored stress

Accumulated or stored stress refers to experiences that may have happened years or even decades ago, that have become stuck in our bodies. As a consequence we would naturally be more hypervigilant in our current lives and more likely to overreact to smaller everyday stressors because our nervous system is already somewhat dysregulated.

In Chapter 2 we looked at adverse childhood experiences and the way they may have impacted our lives. If we have any kind of stored trauma stemming from the past, or there were times when our stress cycle wasn't fully completed, our amygdala will be hypervigilant and primed to expect threat and danger, as opposed to someone's who hasn't had these experiences.

The consequence of this is that we will move out of baseline or our thrive state and activate our stress response quicker than others. Or we may never truly get to experience what a calm baseline really feels like. In our daily lives this shows up as us having less resilience, feeling more 'triggered' by small events and less able to deal with them rationally. This was me all over – getting triggered left, right and centre by small incidental events that created huge turmoil in my body, such as a friend not replying quickly enough to a text or my husband making a flippant joke about my cooking. I was always ready to explode and always feeling agitated. This explains why many people with stored stress turn to alcohol so readily, as it quickly moves us out of the dysregulated, heightened state that we have become stuck in. And as we have already discussed, people with four or more adverse childhood experiences are seven times more likely to develop alcohol use disorder.

We also know that trauma can be stored in different parts of our body. It's not just in our brains where we store traumatic memories but also in our cells and tissues as well. This means the trauma leaves an imprint on our entire body, so it makes sense to work with the body as well as the brain to facilitate healing. In his book *The Body Keeps the Score*, doctor and trauma expert Bessel van der Kolk says:

> We have learned that trauma is not just an event that took place sometime in the past; it is also the imprint left by that experience on mind, brain, and body. This imprint has ongoing consequences for how the human organism manages to survive in the present.

To assess if your nervous system dysregulation began early in life, we can consider a little more of what we discussed in Chapter 2 when we explored events and experiences that we may have suppressed at a young age. We can also look at the nervous systems of our primary caregivers, and the impact this had on how we felt growing up. You may want to only do this deeper work with a therapist. (I did.)

In Chapter 2 we also discussed 'Big T' and 'Little T' events that may have occurred in early life and how they could lead to ongoing issues later on. Remember it's not always the obvious traumatic (Big T) issues that can cause early nervous system dysregulation. It can be bullying, parents in an unhappy marriage with lots of arguing and tension in the family home, moving school and constantly having to make new friends, the death of a pet which was brushed aside, a teacher or sports coach who made us feel inadequate or ashamed.

Trauma can stem from any event that impacted us that we weren't fully supported through, events that were brushed aside as we were told 'Don't be silly' or 'You'll get over it' or that were simply ignored and not mentioned. Perhaps we didn't even tell our parents and we carried these experiences ourselves in our own little bodies. This was certainly my own experience. However, this was not because our parents didn't love us but because they simply didn't know how important this physical processing was as there were so few resources and such little information available at that time. We also have to remember that some of us grew up with parents who were children of the war generation, where any issues outside of having enough food to eat, clothes to wear and a roof over their heads were deemed insignificant.

Studies also show that if our mother was experiencing stress while we were in utero or in the very early years of our life, we are more likely to have a more dysregulated nervous system ourselves. Again, this isn't about blaming a mother who was in this state but understanding where our own nervous system dysregulation may have come from. Did you have a parent who was unpredictable, anxious, on edge and dysregulated themselves? When you were growing up, did you feel calm and relaxed or did you often feel tension and worry? Have you experienced the symptoms of sympathetic dominance for many years?

If we haven't processed these events or feelings effectively, they can lead to nervous system dysregulation that impacts us through our adult years. We just don't even realise it because it's simply our own version of 'normal'. Many of my clients have never experienced a calm baseline and, once they start working on nervous system regulation practices, it can initially feel very foreign.

We've become so comfortable always being 'on' and often feeling tense, alert and anxious that this becomes our new normal. But it's not normal. And as we've learnt, it's not healthy for us long-term as the resulting dysregulation, no matter how big or small, has stayed trapped in our bodies causing all the symptoms previously listed and, in many cases, driven us to drink more. This is why working on releasing stored trauma and developing nervous system flexibility is so important to remove our need for alcohol.

> When we embark on nervous system regulation work, we release the stored trauma in the body which then means we aren't so aggressively triggered by these past events in our present lives.

LET'S REFLECT

On a scale of one to ten, if one is having no stored stress and ten is clearly recognising how much stored stress you have accumulated that is showing up in your daily life, consider where you sit on this scale.

*PLEASE NOTE: If anything uncomfortable or difficult comes up for you in answering these questions, please do seek professional help. I did and it was the greatest act of self-care I've ever shown myself.

Increasing our window of tolerance

If we have any kind of nervous system dysregulation or if we're stuck in the fight/flight or freeze state, it's likely that we will have a very narrow 'window of tolerance'. This term, coined by Dan Siegel, author and Clinical Professor of Psychiatry at the UCLA School of Medicine, describes the window in which we can function and manage our daily stress without getting overly triggered.

People with a healthy, flexible nervous system have a large window of tolerance. This means they can utilise the energy of the fight/flight or freeze response when they need to, but return to baseline and the parasympathetic state quickly. Those who experience constant, chronic stress or have a background of trauma will have a much smaller window, meaning they are triggered and activated more often into the fight/flight or freeze response. My window of tolerance was about a millimetre wide when I started working on my nervous system (my poor husband!). I'm happy to tell you it's grown enormously and I am now calmer, happier and so much more in control of my emotions. You can achieve this too.

It's also important to note that not everyone with a small window of tolerance has specific stored trauma from childhood. For some, our window of tolerance has become smaller and smaller with the pressure and build-up of everyday stressors like work, poor diet, lack of sleep, never-ending lists and always being 'on' in some way.

The below diagram illustrates some ways you can move from fight/flight (hyper arousal) or freeze (hypo arousal) state back to your window of tolerance.

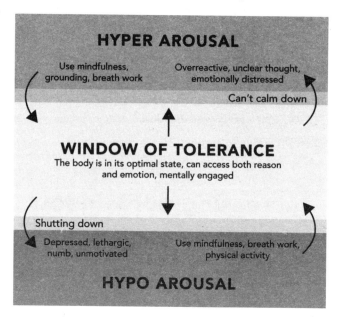

And remember, the goal is not to remove all stressors from your life – that's impossible! The goal is to increase your window of tolerance to cope better with the stress we do have.

The goal isn't to NEVER struggle. The goal is to struggle WELL.

Our path to releasing the stored trauma and nervous system dysregulation of the past and increasing our window of tolerance is a two-fold approach. We can begin to work with our body to release stored trauma (known as somatic therapy – more on this in a moment) and we can take small, practical steps that will increase our tolerance window to improve our mental, physical and emotional wellbeing. Below are some examples of practical steps that can be incorporated into our daily lives.

EXERCISE: SIMPLE SWAPS THAT HAVE BIG IMPACT

Let's look at some everyday swaps of our actions and behaviours that will help us increase our window of tolerance and engage our parasympathetic state whenever we feel ourselves becoming dysregulated.

First reflect on the list you came up with earlier for the daily stressors in your current life.

Consider how you could address each one. I've suggested some possible scenarios in the box below with some example swaps and ideas for change.

Identify which would be helpful for you, as well as adding your own, then commit to trying one swap for the week ahead.

STRESSOR	TIP FOR CHANGE
Reach for phone on waking and go down the 'scroll hole' first thing in the morning, making everything else a rush.	Create a morning routine which includes quiet reflection time, meditation, journaling and silence, with a set time that you check your phone.
Last-minute rush every morning to get breakfast for the family and make lunches for school.	Prepare lunches the night before, lay out breakfast items before bed for children to make own breakfast and ask them to clear away their own dishes.

STRESSOR	TIP FOR CHANGE
Drink too much caffeine and eat too much processed food, which makes us anxious and feel more stressed.	Start the day with hot water and lemon, eat a nourishing breakfast (protein, good-quality fats and whole grains) and have coffee after food (less anxiety inducing).
Back-to-back work meetings and to-do list at work, eating lunch at desk, with no time outside.	Schedule fifteen minutes in the middle of the day to get away from your desk, go for a walk or sit in a quiet spot listening to a meditation. (I have clients who do this in the loo sometimes and say it really helps!)
No time to exercise.	Get up twenty minutes earlier to go for a walk, walk at lunchtime or schedule exercise while kids are at activities. Look for solutions instead of problems.
Struggle to switch off at night.	Start the day with morning sunlight, end it with an Epsom salts bath (magnesium is great for relieving stress) or meditation, turn phone and/or TV off by a certain time.
Living on autopilot, going from one task to the next with little time to self-connect.	Download a reminder app (I use 'Mind Jogger') and add a notification every 90 minutes to take a few deep breaths and walk around to stretch out your body. Ask yourself, 'How do I feel, what do I need?'

Releasing stored trauma with somatic therapy

Peter Levine, author and doctor in medical biophysics and psychology, is often described as the godfather of 'somatic experiencing', also known as somatic therapy. Somatic therapy involves working with the body, rather than the brain (as in cognitive, talking therapy) to release stored trauma and begin to regulate the nervous system.

In talking therapy, known as a top-down approach, we are working with the brain to cognitively understand what may have caused us to experience trauma or an adverse situation that is affecting us. In somatic therapy, a bottom-up approach is used, working with the body to release any stored trauma or fight or flight energy that has become stuck in our nervous system so we begin to feel more soothed, calm and regulated.

There are a couple of techniques in somatic therapy I have personally found beneficial.

BREATHWORK

Breathwork has hands-down been the most effective way for me to release my stored trauma and soothe my nervous system dysregulation. When we are in fight or flight mode, our breathing becomes short and fast. When we slow down our breathing, taking a longer, slower breath out than we breath in, we immediately activate the parasympathetic nervous system.

But breathwork can go much deeper than this and has become a healing modality in itself. By the time I first visited Sharon Jennings, a breathwork facilitator and professional member of the Australian Breathwork Association, I'd been in talk therapy for three years and had made huge progress towards understanding why I was living in sympathetic dominance (and why I had been using alcohol the way I had).

But while I understood all this cognitively, my body was still favouring the fight or flight response and I was still living in that constant hypervigilance. Discovering Sharon was my first step to changing this.

In my first one-to-one session with Sharon, I lay on a mat concentrating only on my breath. I slowly began to relax and sink into the process.

I slipped past my conscious thoughts of 'What am I supposed to be doing? Am I doing it right?' to a deeper place in my subconscious I'd never entered before. In this trance-like, semi-conscious state, I was able to connect to a deeper part of myself in the most profound way. I cried deep, gut-wrenching sobs as old hurts and feelings came up and were released. I hugged myself and released the need to hold on, to always pretend everything was 'fine'. I let myself be ME. I thrashed a little and discharged excess energy through my legs (a common somatic response) and while it sounds crazy as I write this now, I felt like I met my deepest most authentic self, who whispered, 'I've got you, you're safe, you will be okay.' It was profound.

When I came back to awareness and Sharon's gentle and soothing voice, I felt something had shifted. I felt more spacious in my body and somehow lighter. I felt a sense of calm, a sense of self-compassion and a sense of self-acceptance I had never experienced before. This sensation stayed with me for the days and weeks that followed. But how? How did this happen just through breath?

As a qualified practitioner, Sharon describes breathwork as:

a continuous connected breathing practice to journey inward that will take you past your conscious mind and into the subconscious, where we are able to deeply listen, unlock and release mental, emotional and physical blocks from your nervous system. The letting go creates a space within, a space where you were once stuck, where you can safely unveil the layers of protection you have built.

Breathwork continues to be one of the most profound, transformational and healing practices I have ever experienced and is a firm non-negotiable in my ongoing journey to maintain nervous system regulation. If you're interested, I have included some resources at the back of the book to help you find a breathwork practitioner near you.

And when seeing Sharon isn't available to me, I get my mat out at home and play some grounding, soothing music while I feel my breath moving in and out of my body, counting in for six and out for eight. This instantly begins to soothe me.

If you don't have access to a practitioner or are on a limited budget there are numerous online sources, YouTube clips and books that can help you form your own practice. I encourage you to try it!

SOMATIC YOGA

Trauma-informed therapy and yoga (also known as somatic yoga) teaches us to connect deeply to ourselves and our bodies, identify how it feels to be calm and regulated, as well as recognise how it feels when we are uncomfortable and moving into an activated state. This embodied awareness is so powerful on our journey of healing and nervous system regulation. When we create this deeper sense of self-awareness we come to recognise immediately when we are moving out of baseline into a fight or flight response and can take steps to move back, when appropriate. Because I had lived in dysregulation for so long, I didn't even know what a calm baseline felt like. Through somatic yoga and breathwork I found it!

I have always wondered why certain yoga poses can cause us to feel a surge of powerful emotions when we enter them. It is not uncommon to see women burst into tears during a yin or somatic yoga class. This is the body releasing stored, activated energy and finding space and freedom. Women often store old traumas in their hips, and certain yoga shapes and poses can release this trauma. This is what somatic yoga teaches us, particularly yin yoga.

Liz McComish is a somatic therapist, integrated trauma healing practitioner and highly experienced yoga teacher who I worked with to teach my body it was safe for me to sit with uncomfortable emotions, rather than automatically reach for a glass of something to calm me down. Teaching my body to feel safe has been absolutely key to all the changes I've been able to make in my life, including removing alcohol.

'Our bodies hold every memory of our lives: happy, sad and everything in between,' explains Liz. 'These memories inform our nervous system of what the world is like. In response to this our mind creates beliefs and narratives to help us understand and manage our experiences. When we work with the nervous system, we can release traumatic body memories and, naturally, your beliefs and narratives change as well.'

THE HEALING POWER OF SOBRIETY

'No anxiety, no overthinking, no obsessive thoughts, no guilt, no embarrassment, no cringing, no doubts, no regrets, and no controlling behaviour. Just calm.'

MICHELLE

'I'm finally getting to know ME. I'm beginning to enjoy all the feelings I feel. Even the hard, scary ones. '

JEN

'The pure joy I have listening to my son plays his guitar.'

TRISH

EMBODIMENT WORK AND 'FELT' RESOURCES

Jay Fields is an educator, coach and author who has taught the principles of embodied social and emotional intelligence (known as polyvagal theory) for twenty years. Working with Jay taught me daily practices that helped me check in with my body and recognise which state of my nervous system I was in at any given moment, as well as a variety of tools to help me move back to baseline more effectively. This piece of work has been so powerful for me – remember the goal is not to avoid the stress response but simply to notice when we are there and get back to our baseline again quickly.

Using these 'felt' resources I have become adept at recognising if I'm entering sympathetic arousal and am able to catch myself before I continue escalating to the point of no return (when I'm so dysregulated and flooded with cortisol and adrenaline that I have no control over my responses, actions or emotions – my poor family!).

A simple check-in practice Jay taught me is to regularly pause during the day, place one hand on your forehead and one on your chest or belly, close your eyes and breathe. Then ask yourself: 'How do I feel? What do I need? Where am I holding tension in my body? Where could I relax a little more?'

You can do this in any moment!

Build your own stress-busting toolkit

While I think it's worthwhile investing in and consulting qualified practitioners to help with accumulated stress and nervous system dysregulation, it's just as important to build your own personal toolkit when it comes to managing stress on a day-to-day basis. None of these suggestions cost a lot either, so they are great if you have limited finances.

I've listed ten of my favourite go-to's that make up my stress-busting toolkit; however, remember we are all unique and like different things. Part of the fun of this work is giving yourself permission to experiment and try something new! Give these a go and see what works for you.

1. MEDITATION

As someone who lived for so long in a dysregulated state, meditation is not something that has come easily to me. But with practice and commitment it has become an essential tool, particularly when I can feel the stress and anxiety increasing as the day goes on.

We know that one 60-meditation increases our GABA levels (the neuro-transmitter that allows us to feel calm and relaxed) by 27 per cent and people who meditate regularly sleep better.

A podcast hosted by Dr Rangan Chatterjee, author and influential British GP, offered the following advice: 'Everyone should meditate for ten minutes a day. For anyone who says they don't have time, they should meditate for an hour a day.' This made me smile as this was totally me. Meditation changes our perception of how busy we are, how stressed we feel and how much pressure we put on ourselves.

I find practising meditation in the morning or after lunch highly effective. For many of my clients, meditating at the end of the day supports their sleep. (Start small, with short five- or six-minute guided meditations.)

There are numerous apps available that can teach you or help you with meditation. One of my faves is 'Insight timer' which is brilliant for an extensive variety of guided meditations varying in length from three to 60 minutes.

2. HAVENING

This is something that I was actually doing without knowing the name for it. It's a somatic practice which involves a very distinctive self-soothing motion.

There are three places on our bodies that we can practise the havening technique: down the front and sides of the face, the tops of the hands, and crossing your arms across your chest and rubbing the opposite arm from shoulder to elbow – something I have always done in times of distress.

I find rubbing any of these three places calms me and brings me down from a dysregulated place. For more information on how to do it search 'havening' on YouTube.

3. YIN YOGA

In my early days of sobriety, I would get in my car every Tuesday and Thursday evening and drive 25 minutes north of the river to an incredible yin yoga studio. This is where my healing first began. As someone who had always needed to be around people, and had always distracted myself with alcohol, shopping or scrolling on my phone, it was the first time in my adult life I learnt to sit with myself in silence. Sometimes I cried all the way home.

Without even realising it, I was already beginning somatic work by allowing myself to 'be'. If a pose was challenging or had an 'edge' to it which I found uncomfortable, I taught myself to sit with it, go slowly and gradually relax into it. I was teaching myself it was okay to be in discomfort.

There are many videos online that demonstrate yin yoga practices for those who don't want to go to a studio or are on a budget, and I highly recommend the YouTube channel 'Yoga with Kassandra' for many free resources.

4. WALKING

'When in doubt, go for a walk' became my motto when I first quit booze. When a craving for alcohol came, when my stress levels began to rise, when I was angry or sad or anything in between, heading out for a walk always helped. Sometimes I listened to music or a podcast and sometimes I walked in complete silence.

I recently interviewed a naturopath on ways to manage cravings of all kinds, whether it be sugar, alcohol or cigarettes, and she gave me a great tip – head out for a walk and count fifteen houses to allow your mind and body to settle.

Once you get to house number fifteen, turn around and begin a slower walk home. For every house you pass on the way back, think of something you appreciate in your life, in the world, in your surroundings. By the time you get to the last house you will feel markedly calmer and more relaxed than when you started. It's hard not to when you are considering all you have to appreciate about your life.

5. ICE BATHS AND SAUNAS

There is much evidence now to suggest the positive impact of cold water therapy on reducing stress. You only have to look at the popularity of practitioners like Wim Hof.

The theory is that by actively seeking out a way to stress yourself in a controlled environment you are teaching your body to handle stressful events, meaning your resilience in daily life improves. Cold water therapy has also been shown to lower cortisol levels in the body and support production of serotonin, as well as increasing levels of dopamine. In fact, Dr Andrew Huberman says that starting your day with cold water therapy increases your dopamine for up to six hours – what's not to love about that?

If you don't have access to the ocean, the simplest way to expose yourself to the cold is in the shower. At the end of your shower, turn the tap to cold for between 10 and 30 seconds and gradually increase that time over a period of weeks.

If you want to take it one step further, I recommend exploring Wim Hof retreats in your local area or seek out practitioners who combine breathwork with cold water therapy – a practice that I absolutely love. I often rotate between cold water therapy and using a sauna, and have developed such a love for the sauna that I used money I had saved from not drinking to buy my own! There is also evidence to suggest that doing hot yoga (yoga in a heated studio) significantly reduces symptoms of depression.

6. ESSENTIAL OILS

Smell is one of the fastest ways to send a message to your brain that you are safe, as well as being closely linked to memory. We can train our brain to link a certain smell to a feeling. For example, you may have an oil you use or even a candle you burn while you are meditating or having a bath and you associate that specific smell with feeling calm and peaceful. We can then carry that essential oil with us through our day, and this is a powerful and quick way of calming ourselves down when we notice we are becoming anxious or that feelings of fight or flight energy are increasing. I use my favourite oil before presentations and speaking at conferences to relax me and this has been a brilliant tool for many of my clients, too.

Discovering and experimenting with essential oils has been a fantastic process for me and one I am now enjoying with my daughter. In the early days, I would always use an essential oil when I was meditating. I now also use oils for sleep. I add three to four drops into my moisturiser after an evening shower and rub across my chest and shoulders.

7. SOUND

Listening to your favourite calming music or attending a sound bath or sound healing event can play an important part in soothing our nervous system at times of stress.

Sound healing works by activating our parasympathetic nervous system and slowing down our breath, heart rate and even our brainwaves to put us into a trance-like state. There are many online sound healing classes available, as well as those in studios.

8. MOVEMENT AND SHAKING

Exercise has become an absolute non-negotiable in my life when it comes to reducing stress, and if for any reason I can't exercise regularly, I notice it in my thoughts, responses and reactions.

But something I have begun doing more recently is a short shaking session at the end of each day ... and my kids love it too! Limb by limb I shake off any feelings of stress that have built up during the day. Remember earlier when we discussed the importance of ending the stress cycle? This is where shaking can be an excellent and effective practice, particularly if we are experiencing a strong feeling of anger. This happened to me recently and I could really feel the adrenaline and cortisol flooding my body. I was so agitated and restless that I couldn't sit still and so I shook it out (and yes, there may have been some vocals that accompanied my movement!). Boy, did I feel better after.

I have included a link at the back of this book to a shaking video, as well as some other trauma-releasing exercises if going for a run or an exercise class isn't available to you.

9. TOUCH

Reflexology, lymphatic massage, kinesiology and reiki are all practices that I have experimented with. These alternative healing therapies can be incredibly helpful for nervous system regulation because they promote whole body healing (working with the body and not just the mind) and also often induce deep relaxation, a way to teach your body what its baseline, non-activated state feels like.

When I enter my regular reflexology centre, I feel myself relax as soon as I step through the door. I leave feeling deeply rested and soothed. And most importantly, I *like* that feeling. I no longer crave the adrenaline and cortisol-induced high energy, and instead seek contentment, calm and relaxation, which these practices all provide for me.

Since learning how important regulation of my nervous system is to my physical health, I don't have any sense of guilt in adding these practices (we will talk more about guilt in a further chapter). I find calling it 'nervous system regulation practice' more effective than 'self-care'.

10. VOO BREATHING AND HUMMING

Humming and voo breath practices tone something called our vagus nerve, a critical component in our nervous system and crucial for nervous system regulation. This is the main nerve of our parasympathetic nervous system which controls specific body functions such as our digestion, heart rate and immune system. While we don't have any direct control over these functions, we can have some impact on our vagus nerve itself, and incorporating vagal toning exercises into our life helps decrease any build-up of stress and anxiety. There are a number of exercises that help us tone our vagus nerve, which helps us increase our window of tolerance and allows for more nervous system flexibility.

Humming and the voo breath are two extremely effective exercises to tone our vagus nerve. Humming doesn't really need any explanation. To try the voo breath, all you have to do is take a deep breath in and, as you exhale, say the word 'voo' which will create a deep vibration in your body and can sound a little like the foghorn on a ship! When you get to the bottom of the breath, take another deep breath in, exhale with a 'voo' and then repeat three more times. I do this when I'm stopped at traffic lights, or in the shower! For more information on the vagus nerve, I highly recommend *Accessing the Healing Power of the Vagus Nerve* by Stanley Rosenberg.

LET'S REFLECT

Over to you! When you look at this list of ten stress-busting tools, which options really stand out for you as something you would like to try or return to?

What do you currently do to soothe your nervous system?

1. _____

2. _____

3. _____

4. _____

What are you going to add in to soothe your nervous system and engage your parasympathetic 'thrive' state?

1. _____

2. _____

3. _____

4. _____

Finally, complete this sentence:

Next time I feel _____ because of _____, I am going to _____ which will allow me to return to my parasympathetic state. This is important to me because _____.

Where to next?

Developing healthy tools and strategies for the stress that shows up in our lives means we manage stress more easily and comfortably, with a speedy return to 'baseline' instead of getting stuck in the stressed state. Remember the goal isn't to *never* have stress. The goal is to have a flexible nervous system that can cope easily with the stressors in our lives, so they pass through us quicker and thus reduce our need to reach for alcohol at the end of the day to switch off and escape.

One of the main barriers I see to reducing stress is that so many of us find it hard to prioritise our own needs, to set boundaries and to ask for help. But none of us are Wonder Woman and we can't do everything ourselves! That's why, in the next chapter, we are going to explore what a boundary is and how to create our own boundaries to free up time, energy and space for ourselves, as well as learn to prioritise what's important to us.

SOBER ACTION STEPS

☐ Consider the list of symptoms of 'sympathetic dominance' and see if you fall into this category.

☐ Consider if you have accumulated stress and/or stored trauma from earlier life experiences.

☐ Experiment with discovering practices and modalities that work for you in engaging your parasympathetic nervous system and healing past dysregulation.

☐ Commit to one swap to lower your everyday stress load.

☐ Understand this work takes time and dedication but can be your ultimate path to healing and freedom from the need for alcohol.

SOBER SISTERS

PAULA

Drinking alcohol was always a feature in my life, except for pregnancies and when my children were very small. However, I worked out, too, and enjoyed running, participating in many fun runs, even completing a half marathon. If it was a social occasion, though, there was always a glass of something in my hand. It masked my insecurities.

It was only in 2020 that I first began to acknowledge I was using alcohol as a stress relief. That year, emotions were high: the pandemic was beginning to rear its ugly head, I started a new job and then my dad died. It was a perfect storm to drown my sorrows. However, I decided instead to start a 28-day alcohol-free challenge. I began to feel the benefits, so I continued.

Then in October 2021 our nineteen-year-old daughter had a golf-ball-sized tumour on her spine, and an eleven-hour surgery to remove most of it. We were in the hospital twelve hours a day during a Covid wave, under immense emotional strain, while also packing up our house to move and supporting our other daughter, aged sixteen.

The day my daughter was discharged from hospital we moved to our new house. This period was a blur of relief, exhaustion and elation. I then had three weeks back at work before the school summer break. In hindsight, that Christmas and summer break was a period of post-trauma response. My days were spent looking after my daughter's needs, sorting out our new home and unpacking boxes, then in the evening, when the girls were in bed, I'd open the wine.

Really, I was numbing myself to all the intense emotions. If I didn't have a drink I wouldn't sleep, but I wasn't sleeping well because of the alcohol, a vicious circle. I was drinking a bottle of wine most nights for several weeks. Even though

I was on holidays I still felt exhausted. Then in late January, my sixteen-year-old daughter said, 'Mum, the wine has to stop. You can't blot everything out with that.'

I'd never felt so ashamed in my life but it was the wake-up call I needed. Work restarted, giving me more structure and focus, and I started going to a local yoga studio and walking the local trails with my dogs. I acknowledged it was understandable to become dependent, as so many do, on an addictive substance. I also realised how much I'd used alcohol as a shield, to give me a false sense of security.

My husband and I are both approaching ten months without alcohol. Personally, I've achieved this milestone by continually doing the work. Life still has its stresses but I've learned to manage them. I recognise and acknowledge things that might set me off and, depending on what they are, reach into my ever-expanding toolkit to alleviate them. Now Fridays might consist of a beach walk, dinner out (maybe with an alcohol-free beer), a movie or a yoga session. While I don't meditate daily, if I don't practise regularly in some form I find myself feeling dysregulated and out of synch. I've also started mat Pilates with my daughter. Some relationships have changed, some people I now don't see. Others have strengthened, particularly with my daughters, and my husband. I'm reconnecting with my son, after a strained three-year period in which there was little contact. This brings me relief, happiness and hope.

This really is what an alcohol-free life has given me, *hope*. Being authentic (a word used so often but so valid) and being true to yourself and your values, having increased self-respect, and respect and gratitude for those around you. Learning to sit with your feelings, no matter how uncomfortable they may make you feel. It's hard to break away from the norm and expected behaviours but it is so worth it.

CHAPTER 5
TIME AND GUILT

The two main stumbling blocks to stopping drinking

I looked around to see if anyone was looking and, satisfied that all family members were absorbed in their own worlds and activities, I snuck into the pantry and reached behind the bottles of olive oil and vinegar for my half-empty bottle of red wine.

With my heart beating fast, I quickly poured a glass and, standing hidden behind the door of the pantry, drank it with the sole purpose being to get that alcohol into my system as quickly as possible to make all the noise in my head stop.

Once I had drained the glass, I poured a fresh one, walked back into the kitchen and resumed duties of chopping veg for dinner, innocently pretending this was my first glass of the evening.

In truth, I was feeling pissed off, resentful, tired and frustrated. There was always so much to do, there was never any time for me and even though I knew deep down that alcohol wasn't the answer, I didn't have another solution. I had just broken three of my cardinal rules. Rule 1: Don't drink on Monday. Rule 2: Don't drink in secret. Rule 3: Don't lie about my drinking.

And just like that, on autopilot without really thinking, I'd watched myself do all the things I knew I didn't want to be doing. But I felt powerless. I couldn't just magic another hour into the day to get through everything I had to do and I couldn't ever seem to find the confidence to say no to all the extra demands. Alcohol, momentarily, made it all stop.

While I knew on a deeper level that drinking wasn't really the answer, I just didn't know where to look to find any other solution. And the thing about alcohol is that because of the big dopamine punch it delivers, we get our feeling of reward while we are doing 'all the things'. It's a way of making ourselves feel just a teeny bit better when we feel like nothing more than glorified chefs, cleaners, waitresses, house maids, Uber drivers and counsellors. Can you relate?

We have talked so much in the previous chapter about stress and the impact it has on our physical health, and why we need to prioritise activities that will soothe our dysregulated nervous systems. Yet the truth is, many of us find it incredibly challenging to actually *do the things we know can help us*, and instead are still relying on an evening wine for solace. Why?

The reality is that so many women carry the lion's share of the household work, while also working long hours, which leaves very little time for ourselves. And we feel guilty about even taking any time for ourselves, as we have been conditioned to believe that 'self-care is selfish'. There are two main barriers I see again and again to reducing our stress and prioritising ourselves: time and guilt.

> **The problem with alcohol is that we can get our reward and relaxant while doing all the other things we need to do and it doesn't involve us taking any time away from the home, the family or the kitchen.**

We can do the ironing, prep dinner, empty the dishwasher and mop the floors with a glass in hand and we don't have to experience the guilt of leaving the home or taking time away from our chores. But if we want to create a life where we don't want or need alcohol at the end of each day (or let's face it, sometimes by 1 p.m.), we have to learn to set boundaries, ring-fence our time and energy, and learn to say no to others and yes to ourselves.

Because what's the alternative? A life of always feeling resentful, pissed off, overwhelmed, exhausted and eventually, ill.

Yes, I know saying no to others can be scary! But when we remove alcohol our clarity, confidence and self-esteem begin to grow, we stop feeling shame about the night before and we start to prioritise ourselves, which leads to us feeling happier and more content. And remember what we've already said – the greatest gift we give to the people we love is our own happiness. A mum, wife or friend who is constantly exhausted, angry or sad isn't supporting this at all.

Are you a human *doing*, *giving* or *being*?

When we live in this never-ending cycle of prioritising everyone else's needs so that we're always at the bottom of our to-do list (meaning we never actually get to us), we become overwhelmed, exhausted and resentful. (Yes, you know it's true!)

We are in danger of becoming a:

- Human *giving* – someone who always gives to everyone else and never to themselves.

- Human *doing* – someone who is always doing 'stuff', but never getting to the end of the list (Are you bored and unfulfilled but always busy? A clear sign you're a human doing.)

But remember you are a:

- Human *being* – someone who needs to be connected to yourself, to be doing things you love that bring you joy.

The sad truth is that for many of us, this is a foreign concept and one we simply can't fathom as being possible in our own lives.

Dr Libby Weaver, one of Australasia's leading nutritional biochemists, encapsulates this perfectly in her book *Rushing Woman's Syndrome*, when she writes: 'Never before have women been in such a hurry to do so many things and be there for so many people.'

We are overwhelmed and run ourselves ragged all day just trying to keep up; the pressure and expectation is intense and the more out of control we feel, the greater desire we have to control everything, meaning we take on more. It's relentless and exhausting and most of us are living like this 24/7.

If you recognise that you oscillate between giving and doing, and spend only a small amount of time in the being category, or none at all, it's no wonder you're reaching for a wine each night!

For many of us, alcohol is the only way we can remove that relentless sense of pressure and urgency.

In my coaching, I ask my clients to complete Gretchen Rubin's 'The Four Tendencies Quiz', which is available on her website. This quiz explores the four core tendencies that we all fall into, and pinpoints which major tendency can be described as our default setting:

- Upholder: loves routine, is organised, meets expectations, likes structure.

- Questioner: always questioning and likes to have all the information before they can decide or commit.

- Rebel: resists authority and values freedom and choice.

- Obliger: puts others before themselves and often 'keeps the peace'.

Obligers are your classic people-pleasers and guess how many of my clients fall into this category? Over 80 per cent! And guess what Obligers have the biggest problem with? Saying no to others in order to put themselves first. (No wonder so many grey area drinkers identify as Obligers.)

Obligers live a life of mostly meeting others' needs and discarding their own, in order not to let anyone down. They would rather disappoint themselves than other people. But what is the impact of living life in this way?

Gabor Maté covers this in detail in his book *The Myth of Normal*. In fact, he dedicates an entire chapter to it called 'Society's shock absorbers: Why women have it worse' which I highly recommend reading. He describes women as being at much higher risk of suffering chronic pain, migraines, fibromyalgia, irritable bowel syndrome and autoimmune conditions like rheumatoid arthritis. He also states that 80 per cent of all people diagnosed with autoimmune conditions are women. This blew my mind! Many of these conditions can be linked to chronic stress and the greater sense of isolation that women are experiencing today, compared to the past. He also notes that rheumatoid arthritis strikes women three times more often than it does men, lupus afflicts women by a disproportionate factor of nine and female-to-male ratio of multiple sclerosis (MS) has been rising for decades. In the 1930s the ratio was 1:1, and today for every male who has MS there are 3.5 women – something Maté says cannot be linked to genetics or diet and instead attributes to the increased stress in women's lives.

Maté labels four character traits more commonly displayed in women (very compatible with the Obliger tendencies) and the impact these have on women's health.

1. We have more emotional concern for the needs of others.

2. We suppress healthy anger. This means we don't feel comfortable expressing anger, even when it is justified, so we keep it held in. Many of us avoid confrontation and this is very detrimental.

3. We identify with duty and responsibility.

4. We believe that we are responsible for other people's emotions and we mustn't disappoint anybody.

Many of these traits are inherent in women. We have been accultured to play a specific role in society. We absorb the stresses of our families and our partners. In his interview with Dr Chatterjee for the podcast 'Feel Better, Live More', Gabor Maté discussed a study in Sweden that showed if a woman was experiencing depression while she was pregnant, that increased the risk of a premature birth at about 32 to 36 weeks. However, if a male was stressed while his partner was pregnant this increased the risk of an even earlier premature birth. Why? Because the woman was absorbing the stress of her partner. As women, we do this without even realising it. Contemporary studies have shown that women took on more emotional stress during the pandemic lockdowns, particularly the stress of their partners and children. It's no wonder we also saw a correlation with a rise in women's drinking during this time. And the fact that alcohol use disorder in women has increased so significantly correlates with the fact women absorb so much of everyone else's stress, as well as their own.

We also have to consider what has been role-modelled to us for years by our mothers, aunts, grandmothers and any other female figures in our lives. It's been our cultural tradition for so long that woman look after everyone else. But we also have to remember that our female ancestors were not also working the hours that we are today while carrying the same amount of pressure, expectation and domestic workload.

What do you think when you consider the character traits Gabor Maté mentions? Do they resonate with you? I am not saying this is wrong or that you need to completely change who you are (these traits are commonplace for women), but I am saying there are steps you can take to create more balance around meeting others' needs *as well as* your own. It doesn't have to be an either/or scenario. It can be both – we can attend to the needs of others and still not put ourselves at the bottom of the to-do list. We get to matter. We get to be important. It's our life, too. We are allowed to make sure we are okay, and to create a life that has meaning and joy for ourselves instead of only focusing on others. It's *essential* to do this if we want to change our drinking.

We can start by looking objectively at our lives and lifestyle choices to see where the changes need to be.

One quote I absolutely love is from Socrates: 'The unexamined life is not worth living.' And there is also this from Bessel van der Kolk in his book *The Body Keeps the Score*: 'As long as one doesn't examine oneself, one is completely subject to whatever one is wired to do, but once you become aware that you have choices, you can exercise those choices.'

This means *you have choices!* Let's begin to live *consciously*, to reflect on and consider our lives, and actively make choices and decisions that benefit us, instead of doing the same thing we've always done and feeling pissed off and resentful that nothing has changed. Remember 'to live' is a verb; it's a practice and a conscious decision to live our lives the way we want, instead of simply existing.

> To create change, to not *need* our evening drink, we
> have to do things differently, and learn to put ourselves
> first – and get out of that damn kitchen!

LET'S REFLECT

How much of your average day is taken up meeting the needs of others, whether it is giving advice to a friend or family member, attending something because you don't want to let anyone down, or listening to your partner download after a particularly difficult day?

How much of your average day is taken up doing things not for your own pleasure but for other people's, like driving kids around, prepping dinner, shopping, working, attending meetings, walking the dog, organising a trip or shopping for family needs?

How much of your average day is spent being with yourself, feeling connected to yourself and doing something for your own pleasure and joy, whether that's a yoga class, reading a book, taking a bath, going to your favourite dance class, gardening or meditating?

The importance of role-modelling

As we have discussed, our female lineage has played a role in the women we grow up to be and the traits that we develop. But up until the current generation, our female ancestors weren't living the life that we have today or the life that our daughters will go on to experience, which involves more juggling, pressure and stress than ever before. I believe it is important to face this full on and understand that in order to live with this stress it is absolutely essential we have practices in place to prevent the chronic illnesses that are becoming more prevalent in women. In doing this, we are role-modelling to the next generation that they don't have to use wine as their only coping strategy, and that there are so many alternative options available to them to support their mental and physical health.

A dear friend of mine said recently, 'I feel I am the worst mother in the world, I leave the house at 7 p.m. every Tuesday and Thursday to play tennis and I'm not home until after the kids are in bed.' I replied, 'Hell no, you're not! In my eyes this makes you the BEST mother in the world! You're modelling to your kids, and especially your daughter, that it's okay for mums to take time for themselves, it's okay for women to do things that make them happy and it's okay for mums to be away from the home.' I don't think there's a stronger message we can give our daughters – we (and therefore they) are allowed to create and live a life that makes us happy and that is full of activities and experiences that are simply for our own joy (more on this in further chapters). If you ever experience guilt over taking time for yourself, consider the message you want to pass on to both your sons and daughters: that women are as entitled as men are to take time away from the home to do things they love.

Check in with your 80-year-old self

In her book *The Top Five Regrets of the Dying*, palliative nurse Bronnie Ware shares the top five regrets of those at the end of their lives. They are:

1. I wish I'd had the courage to live a life true to myself, not the life others expected of me.

2. I wish I hadn't worked so hard.

3. I wish I'd had the courage to express my feelings.

4. I wish I'd stayed in touch with my friends.

5. I wish I'd let myself be happier.

What do you feel when you read this? This list impacted me significantly and was vital in my decision to make significant changes to how I lived my life. I like to reflect on these regrets and ask myself regularly: 'Am I acting in a way that my 80-year-old self would be proud of?'

When I'm going through a difficult time or have tough decisions to make, I check in with my imagined 80-year-old self. 'What would *you* have me do?' I ask her 'What would you want for me in this moment?' She nearly always has the answer. One of her most repeated responses is:

'Slow down, it's not a race, enjoy the ride instead of always striving for the destination.' Asking her this question also supports me in feeling less guilty when I make choices that are for me. Because I remember that I'm doing this for her, too.

So many people I see wait for there to be a major catastrophe in their life – an illness, an almost fatal crash, the death of a loved one – before they make the decision to live differently. But you don't have to wait for that awful event. You can choose to live differently now. Today. Don't wait a moment longer!

Write down what your 80-year-old self would wish for you. Consider how aligned your life is to that wish right now.

My 80-year-old self would wish that I changed _____ so that I created a life with more _____ which is important to me because _____.

Choose to do it differently

Rarely do we see anyone in our world smashing goals and making huge, positive life changes when they're hungover, tired and anxious each day. Alcohol prevents us from living up to our full potential. It prevents us from creating the wonderful, big, fulfilling life we all desire. The very one we've just written down we want to live!

But remember, it is your responsibility and no one else's. There isn't going to be someone charging in on a white horse to magically change your life and make it how you want it. It's entirely up to you. Don't wait for opportunities to come to you. Create your own! It's time! Are you with me?

As one of Australia's leading motivational speakers, author Craig Harper, often says: 'Your life will not accidentally end up awesome. Make the choice, find the courage, do the work.' That means putting yourself first and living by the mantra: 'I get to matter.'

> The first real step to doing things differently is to create a life your 80-year-old self will be proud of.

The benefit of boundaries

When I first quit alcohol, I had no idea what a boundary was, let alone how to set one. As someone who craved connection, friendship and the need to fit in, saying 'no' to something or someone felt alien and counter-intuitive. *'Surely if I say no, people won't like me anymore. Maybe they won't want to be my friend and then I will be lonely and always left out, right?'*

Yet by learning to set boundaries, I actually created more free time, allowed my nervous system to settle, improved my mental wellbeing and mindset, and enabled myself to be more present for the people and things that matter most to me. I've also created deeper and more authentic connections with the people I love and, most importantly, with myself. I know myself. I trust myself. I love myself. What's not to love about that?

I consider boundaries to be the mental, physical, emotional and financial walls I put up to defend myself. They are a way to protect my time and energy, and prevent me from entering nervous system dysregulation. They are also a way of showing others how I want and need to be treated. Oprah Winfrey has a famous quote about boundaries: 'You have to be able to set boundaries, otherwise the rest of the world is telling you who you are and what you should be doing.'

There are absolutely no negatives to setting boundaries other than it may upset the people who benefit from you having none! Yes, one of the key reasons we don't set boundaries is our fear of letting others down.

The sad truth is that so many of us would rather disappoint ourselves than disappoint others. We fear that we are being mean or letting others down if we say 'no' and, for many of us, our way of feeling 'good enough', our coping mechanism for feeling good about ourselves, is in doing things for others. So, if we stop doing that, where do we get our self-worth from? Let me tell you – we get it from setting boundaries, healing our past and creating deeper self-connection, all of which we are exploring in this book. When we love ourselves, we don't have to give to others all the time to feel 'enough', because we already do.

Yes, there will be resistance from other people at first. Especially from those who don't want us to change, because it suits them better if we stay the same. And while it does feel uncomfortable at first, there are ways of doing it that make it easier.

Recently a dear friend asked me: 'Do you ever daydream about being involved in an accident, nothing so bad that it's life-changing, but enough to put you in hospital for a few days where someone is just looking after you, feeding you and checking on you and no one expects anything from you?' If this scenario is something that you daydream about, take it as a sure sign that it's time to start setting boundaries today!

When we don't have boundaries we are basically on call to meet everyone else's needs apart from our own, which as we know from Chapter 4, leads to burnout and nervous system dysregulation and, as we've just discussed, can also lead to chronic illness.

The benefit to setting boundaries is that we begin to feel calmer, more regulated and in control of what is happening, have healthier relationships that bring us more joy, and experience more presence and connection in our lives.

So how do we set boundaries?

The best way to describe how a boundary works is to think about drawing an imaginary circle around yourself.

Inside your circle are behaviours, activities and actions that make you feel good. Outside the circle are those that do not.

Our boundaries are not just a way of managing our own time and behaviours, they also teach other people in our lives to respect us and how we want to be treated. They are a line to separate where you end and another person begins.

I have realised that the people I respect the most in my life are those with the clearest boundaries!

When it comes to setting boundaries, there are five key areas in life you can look at. And believe me, doing this work is so important to remove our incessant desire to switch off with alcohol at the end of each stressful, exhausting day.

The five key areas are:

1. Work

2. Friendships

3. Family

4. Relationships

5. Self

A clue to working out where you most need a boundary is to consider these five areas and reflect on which one you find yourself complaining about the most. That's where you need your first boundary.

1. WORK

When it comes to work, remember that people will treat you according to the boundaries you create and act upon. We can't say we are sick of getting emails at 7 p.m. if we keep answering them, as by replying, all we are doing is telling our colleagues we are online and available.

My friend often moaned that she was the one her boss emailed on a Saturday and not her colleague. I asked her if her colleague answered emails on the weekend and she said, 'No – she never checks her phone at weekends.' Case proven!

People will take advantage of our good nature where they can. Create a boundary, communicate it and stick to it!

Circle which of these could help you set a boundary at work.

- I only check emails up until 6 p.m. and then my phone goes off until 8 a.m.

- I don't engage in office gossip and if someone tries to draw me into a conversation, I say it's not something I'm comfortable talking about or I change the subject.

- I don't check my work emails on holiday or at the weekends.

- I ask for help when I feel overloaded or at capacity.

- I ask to be paid commensurately with my job.

THE IMPACT OF MY SOBRIETY

'I see my value in my world and
I know what I deserve.'

KATE

'I laugh so much more, and can
handle daily anxiety and general life
stuff so much better, and I let things
go easier.'

BRIDGET

'The unexpected benefit is how
much happier I am.'

DIDDI

2. FRIENDSHIPS

My all-time favourite saying when it comes to friendships and boundaries is 'You can't keep getting mad at people for sucking the life out of you if you keep giving them the straw.'

When it comes to friendships, we have to stop giving people the bloody straw!

Many of us have slipped into roles in our friendships which may have been established years ago and we become the person who is known for that thing – whether it is the one who listens, the one who always helps, the one with practical advice, or the one who drinks and parties.

Establishing boundaries in long-term friendships can feel uncomfortable at first, especially if you've been placed in a role that others have become accustomed to, but it can be done with love and without needing to offend or hurt the other person.

In healthy friendships, we are mutually supportive of each other, we trust each other, we can talk authentically about our feelings, our friends respect our time and energy, and the friendship can evolve and grow as we do. Our friends support us and the decisions we make to improve our lives.

In unhealthy friendships we notice our friend takes more than gives, talks more than listens or is unsupportive when we want to change. We may also realise we don't have anything in common but stay in the friendship out of duty.

Circle which of the statements below could help you set a boundary with your friends.

- 'I can't talk this evening. If it isn't urgent, I will call you tomorrow when I have more time.'

- 'I love supporting you as much as possible, but feel I am offering you a lot of advice that you aren't taking or listening to. It's draining for me to have the same conversations and to feel like your dumping ground for all your difficulties. I am happy to help but if you don't want solutions or support, I think it best we don't talk about this.'

- 'I'm feeling sad and uncomfortable that you aren't being more supportive of my decision to remove alcohol. It's a really big decision for me and one I haven't taken lightly, and your support means the world.' (Spoiler alert – lots more on this in the next chapter!)

- 'Sunday is a family day for me so I'm not free to catch up, even though I know it's more convenient for you. How about next Friday evening?'

3. FAMILY

Whether it's our parents or our kids, this is where the boundary line can become really blurred, and where we often have to work the hardest to set boundaries.

Our parents may feel we 'owe' them something in their later years and expect us to drop everything the moment they phone, or our kids think they have access to our time and energy 24/7.

Setting boundaries in this area can free up so much of our time and energy.

Both of the statements below could help you set a healthy boundary with your family.

- 'Mum, I'm not available to speak to you every night at 6 p.m. as it's a difficult time when I get home from work and I'm rushing around after the kids. I would like to move our calls to Wednesday and Sunday at 7 p.m. when I can give you more of my time and energy.'

- 'Kids, you are old enough to take on some responsibility for household chores. Let's work together to see what some of those chores could be.' (I did this with my kids when they were seven and nine. It worked!)

EXERCISE: HOW TO WORK OUT WHO DOES WHAT IN THE FAMILY

My own coach Ali taught me this exercise and I absolutely love it! Hold a family meeting and on a piece of paper create a column for everyone in the house. Then ask everyone to write in their column the jobs they do to ensure the house runs smoothly.

For kids it might be 'feed the dog', 'empty the dishwasher', 'bring in the washing'. Then you start writing everything you do in your column. It can be an eye-opening exercise for everyone in the house to see what you actually do on a daily and weekly basis and often creates a newfound respect for your role and all you juggle.

Then ask everyone to consider what they can take off your list and add onto their list. Ensure this list is pinned up where everyone can see it, so all members of the home are fully aware of their own responsibilities.

The time you will get back and the arguments you will prevent from completing this exercise are priceless!

---

4. RELATIONSHIPS

Establishing boundaries in our romantic relationships is a major step towards creating a healthy relationship. However, most of us never talk about this and we simply put up with how things are for fear of confrontation or argument.

One of the most effective steps to creating healthy boundaries in a relationship is to identify what your needs are. We all have different needs based on our upbringing, our love languages and our relationship history but if we don't communicate these to our partners, we can end up angry and resentful. But here's the thing – they aren't mind-readers! Not only do we have to understand our needs, we also need to communicate them.

Below are some example statements that can help you set a boundary in your relationship.

- 'It's important to me that we have an equal distribution of household chores. I would love if we could draw up a list of chores at the start of each week and delegate accordingly.'

- 'I really love it when you give me a hug and kiss when you get home from work and ask me how my day was.'

- 'Before launching into a big topic that you really want to talk about, can you ask me if it's a good time or give me advance notice so I can think about it beforehand.'

- It's important to me we both have time to enjoy individual activities that we each love. Let's sit down with the diary and work out when we can each have some time to ourselves outside of the family.

5. SELF

This may be the most important place we can set boundaries – and the hardest!

Most of us moan about having no time to do things like yoga, meditation, exercise or explore a new hobby, and yet our screen time can average three hours a day! Start considering where you need to set boundaries for yourself to allow for more time and energy to do things you love that bring you joy.

Have an honest conversation with yourself about what you would like to improve in your life and the boundaries you can set to make this happen. I have used some examples from my own life below:

- I limit my screen time to 90 minutes a day. I check it for 45 minutes in the morning and 45 minutes in the evening. I use an app blocker to enforce this.

- I put 10 per cent of my income into a savings account to use each month for activities and experiences that bring me joy. (I did this with the money I saved not drinking. I had enough to buy an infrared sauna for my garden and a peloton bike!)

- I prioritise eating nutritious and healthy foods that nourish my body and provide lasting energy so that I can get the most out of my days and feel the best I can.

- I have a morning routine that sets me up for the day and follows a process of reflection, affirmations, meditation and movement.

EXERCISE: GIVE YOURSELF PERMISSION

Out of the five areas in life where you may struggle with boundaries – work, friendships, family, relationships, self – identify the one you complain about the most. Now we can work on establishing your first boundary. The benefit of doing this is that we free up time for ourselves.

Next, decide to give yourself full permission to establish that boundary. Ensure to record your daily win at the end of each day as this is an essential part of the process. This could be by ticking off something in a journal or, when brushing your teeth at night, reflecting on what went well today and considering what you're proud of.

Next, complete this sentence:

The boundary I am going to set is _____. The impact of setting this boundary will allow me to _____. This is important to me because _____. I will start by setting myself this goal of _____ and I will congratulate myself by ticking it off in my journal each day I complete it.

Identifying your needs

NEWSFLASH: You can meet your own needs without making others unhappy.

A major part in the journey of self-discovery is understanding and then being able to meet our own needs, something I couldn't do when I was drinking. I didn't even know what my needs were beyond the next drink. The process of setting boundaries means we become able to identify and understand our own needs in a range of situations and relationships. It is a major step in the process of removing the need for alcohol from our lives.

In therapy, when I was first asked the question: 'Are your needs being met?' I had no idea because I didn't even know what my needs were, let alone how to go about meeting them. This is where the exercise that life coach and educator Jay Fields gave me has really made a difference.

To determine my need at any given moment, I take a moment to myself, place one hand on my forehead and one hand on my heart, close my eyes and ask myself: 'How do I feel, what do I need?' It's incredible the responses I find myself offering. 'I feel thirsty, I need a drink. I feel tired, I need to lie down. I feel restless, I need to move my body. I feel sad, I need a hug. I feel disconnected, I need to speak to a friend. I feel overwhelmed, I need to take some deep breaths.' This exercise is so simple and yet so effective in many ways – it supports us to truly understand that we are *allowed* to have needs, and it supports us to find a way for our needs to be met, whether that's asking someone for something or meeting that need ourselves.

I know that asking for a need to be met, even from loved ones, can be very tricky. Perhaps you, like me, also have a strong belief that it's weak to ask for help. Perhaps you have always valued independence and self-reliance and it makes you uncomfortable to ask for help or ask for what you need. But if we don't start doing things differently, we stay stuck. We stay in the old patterns that haven't been working.

EXERCISE: ASSESS YOUR NEEDS

We can start by thinking about different areas of our life, what our needs are in that area and if they are being met.

For example, at work I need to feel respected, validated, recognised, fairly treated, encouraged, empowered and fulfilled.

In my friendships I need to feel supported, accepted, cared for, safe, loved and listened to.

In my relationship I need to feel seen, appreciated, desired, cared for, loved, safe, trusted and understood.

1. Work

2. Friendships

3. Family

4. Relationships

Choose one area of your life to complete this sentence.

I have recognised that my need(s) in this area of my life are: _____. I will take a step towards having this need met by _____. This is important to me because _____. When this need is being met, I will feel _____.

It's time to be brave and voice our needs! The moment I started doing this was the moment my relationships and my life really began to change.

Adding to your bucket

Once we have established a practice of setting a boundary, understood that taking time for ourselves is essential and not selfish and begun asking for our needs to be met, we will have more time and/or mental headspace, which means more energy. And with this new time and energy, we can start adding *in* to our lives.

I like to think of my mental, physical and emotional energy in terms of a big bucket. When we wake in the morning, generally speaking, our bucket is full (provided we've had a great sleep, hence the importance of prioritising what time we go to bed and a before-bed sleep routine).

Over the course of the day, events and actions occur that begin to deplete that bucket: we exercise, we multitask a million things at once, we commute in peak-hour traffic, we don't have time to eat well, we have a super busy day at work, we have to rush to get the kids to activities, we try and squeeze in chats to friends while driving from A to B, we might have to finish work at home that evening as we left early … By the time it gets to 5 p.m. our energy bucket is empty, with nothing to sustain us through a few more hours of being needed and being 'on'.

And this is why all good intentions of not drinking that day often fall by the wayside as all our energy is MIA.

We need to find ways to add in energy boosters and remove energy drains.

To ensure our bucket isn't empty by the end of the day, we have to consider what to add *in* through the day to keep topping up our depleting energy levels. Because we don't have a limitless supply of energy, after all.

We can't constantly live our lives at ten-out-of-ten capacity because then the smallest of things sends us over the edge. We need to find ways through the day to get that capacity level down.

We can add in energy boosters in a variety of ways, such as:

- Set a reminder on your phone to get up and go for a walk every couple of hours to clear your head, perhaps listening to a walking meditation.

- Put on soothing music in the car when you're driving and use a relaxing essential oil at the same time.

- Yoga nidra: This is my go-to restorative meditation that has seen me through so many exhausting days. They say twenty minutes of yoga nidra is the equivalent of two hours deep sleep. (Info in the resources section.)

- Never underestimate the power of your breath to engage the parasympathetic nervous system and calm you down, as discussed in Chapter 4.

- Try a fifteen-minute meditation instead of scrolling on your phone when you're waiting for the train or the kids to finish an activity.

- Eating healthy and energising food to sustain energy through the day.

- Plan an activity every day just for you, no matter how small.

- Start your day by journaling your responses to the question: 'How am I showing myself love and topping up my energy today?'

Which of these could you choose as a goal to start working on?

Set small goals

James Clear's book *Atomic Habits* is the bible for creating new habits and a book I highly recommend. He describes a method called 'Implementation intention'. This means we set a goal that includes precise detail of *what* we are doing and *when* we are doing it.

So instead of setting goals such as 'eat healthily' or 'exercise' we need to get really clear on what we mean. So we might say: 'I will eat six different vegetables and two pieces of fruit a day, only consuming sugar and processed food in one meal at the weekend and drinking 2 litres of water a day.'

For 'exercise' we might say 'I am going to the gym at 6 a.m. Monday, Wednesday and Friday, walking at 6 p.m. on Tuesday and Thursday and going to the 8 a.m. yoga class every Sunday.' When we are really clear with the goals we are setting we are more likely to stick to them. This increases our sense of pride and wellbeing and we are more likely to continue these new habits.

We can also apply the practice of implementation intention for setting boundaries.

LET'S REFLECT

What is one goal you want to set for yourself for the next week in relation to a boundary, prioritising time or an activity for you?

I am going to _____ at _____ on _____. This is important to me because _____.

Commit to stick

One thing I know for sure is that you must be 100 per cent committed to doing this work and you have to follow it through. You can't communicate a boundary and then not follow through as this indicates to others that you are not serious and then you'll continue to find boundaries being blurred and people taking advantage of your goodwill.

Communicating the boundary, sticking to it and then adding in something for you to replace the old behaviour is the secret to establishing long-term change.

Remember, too, our new activity is our *reward* for setting the boundary instead of relying on alcohol to help us cope with a boundary-less life. Giving ourselves permission to set boundaries to free up some time and not feel guilty about this is the key to prioritising ourselves more.

We've talked a lot in this chapter about the boundaries we can set with other people. This is an important process of preserving our time and energy and also removing the pressure to drink. But does this mean having to completely change our friendship group? And what on earth do we do if our partner still drinks? This is exactly what we are going to explore next.

SOBER ACTION STEPS

☐ Recognise if you are a human doing, human giving or human being.

☐ Consider what you would like to be different in your life in regard to work, family, friends and relationships. Visualise the person you want to become.

☐ Choose one of the areas mentioned above where you want to set a boundary.

☐ Identify the needs you have in that area of your life.

☐ Set the boundary and/or ask for a need to be met.

☐ Set a goal and once that goal has become your habit, move onto the next area. Remember – there is no rush! This is the rest of your life.

DONNA

I had done alcohol-free challenges before and felt great while on them but always returned to drinking. One night I had had a bottle of wine and felt it had really no effect. The following day my sixteen-year-old daughter asked if I remembered the conversation we'd had and I had no idea what she was talking about. Her face was enough for me to know that if I wanted to have any valuable relationship with my kids then it was time to have a break. It was then I floated the idea with friends and my husband that I wanted to embark on a 'year of health'. However, in my mind, I knew it meant trying a life without alcohol. Everyone thought it was a great idea and I heard lots of 'Yeah, I should do that.' I was the only one who did.

So far, I am seventeen months in and my life has completely changed for the better. I have dropped 12 kilos and kept it off. My diet is healthy and I now have more energy. My relationships with my kids are better than I could have ever imagined and I no longer feel 'the fear' or anxiety like I used to after a night of drinking.

I have a 'toolbox' that works for me. I walk the dogs every day and do yoga every morning, meditation and fasting. I peruse menus before I go out to check for any mocktails on offer. I occasionally have a non-alcoholic beer if I feel I need to be more part of the group but generally I no longer feel that I am missing out. I regularly ask myself: 'If I eat or drink this, what's in it for me?'

Being alcohol-free has enabled me to dig deep to find out who I really am and do you know what? I like who I am. I may not be the last person standing at the end of the party anymore but I am the first to get up the following morning and that makes me feel good about myself. I have learnt not to people-please anymore and my new favourite line (which my family is sick of hearing) is, 'I'm not available for that.'

I know that when I engage in positive self-care, I am a better wife, mother and colleague. I say this as I sit in a wellness and yoga retreat while the family are at home. Nothing but me doing good stuff for myself and I don't feel any guilt at all.

It's now all about being present in my daily life, feeling an overwhelming sense of gratitude for what I have and trying to be the best person I can be for me.

CHAPTER 6
SOBER LOVE
Navigating our romantic relationships

I met Gus at the ripe age of 24, while I was backpacking around Australia. I booked a trip from Perth to Broome on one of the backpackers 'hop on, hop off' buses and guess who was the bus driver/tour guide? Yep, there he was in all his cute Kiwi glory. Thinking I was playing it cool, I approached him that evening at the backpackers with the very classy line of, 'Hey, wanna come and play a drinking game?' When a relationship starts with one of you asking the other to down tequila shots, it kind of sets the tone for the years ahead, right?

We partied together around the world, from Perth to London to New York to Croatia to Miami, in the true hedonistic style of young, carefree adults earning their own money for the first time, with no ties or responsibilities.

While there may have been some whispers among my friends that we were very 'different' (after all, he grew up on a farm in rural New Zealand and rode a horse to school, and I was a true city girl who didn't travel anywhere without a hairdryer, heels and make-up), it never occurred to me that this might end up being a problem. And honestly it wasn't. Because at that time, partying and drinking were our number one priorities and we both excelled at them.

We never judged each other for our drinking, we never criticised each other's drinking and we never thought it was a problem. Partying and alcohol were the glue that tied us together. It was our thing. We thought alcohol would stay our shared hobby into retirement when we planned to travel the world, cab sav in hand. Who would have thought any different in your 20s?

Given the number of women I've coached over the years who've struggled with their relationship during sobriety, this early mutual love of alcohol is a pretty common story. And it begs the question: what happens to your relationship if you take alcohol out of the equation?

A new foundation

I'm sure you've all cried: 'My partner just doesn't understand me!' at some point in your life, but when you choose to stop drinking it can become a real point of tension in relationships, of all different shapes and sizes.

When I stopped drinking, I remember feeling so alone and confused, like Gus and I were on completely different levels. I was on a path of reflection and awareness, gobbling up all the information I could on alcohol, sobriety, gut health, managing emotions and everything in between while he still came home and cracked a beer every night, like we always used to do together. It was confronting and, in all honesty, really scary. All I could think was, 'What if we never reconnect from this, what if it means our marriage is over?' It is really common to feel this way when we start making changes in our life but our partner isn't doing the same.

When you've spent a lot of time drinking together in a partnership or friendship (regardless of your sexual orientation or preferences) and one of you decides to quit alcohol, it can cause you to question a lot of things – including the very foundation your partnership was built on. Equally, if you're single, then you'll start to question what you should be looking for in a partner. For example, do they need to be a non-drinker too? (We will be covering more on this topic later.)

If alcohol has been significant in your life and/or relationship and even been a way of connecting, then removing it is going to have a big impact.

Week in, week out I receive emails and messages from women asking how to deal with this shift and sharing the confusion and isolation it has created. There will be times when you notice the foundations of your relationship feel less stable and more rocky and you may begin to feel unsettled, fearful about the future or disconnected from your partner. This is all very normal but the biggest issue I see is that we don't prepare for it or expect it, so we aren't equipped to deal with it.

So how *do* we do this?

> Initially, it's really important we remember that this is *your* decision not to drink, and not theirs.

It's your story, not theirs

The decision to stop drinking is not something to be pushed onto someone else. This is something we are choosing to do for us and it's not fair to expect them to join us. If you decided to take up tap dancing, I can't imagine you would insist your partner join you. If you chose to stop eating meat or sugar, I can't see that you would insist your partner do it, too. It's the same with alcohol.

In my experience of coaching thousands of women to remove alcohol from their lives, one thing I know for sure is that you have to *want* to quit for it to work. It rarely succeeds if you're doing it to make someone else happy or it's under duress. If your partner doesn't want to quit drinking, it's not your place to tell them they should.

Even if we think or suspect that our partner is using alcohol in a dysfunctional way, it is not our place to tell them they need to quit. (The exception in this case would be if your partner's drinking is having a negative effect, physically, emotionally and even financially, on the family. Then it would be a good idea to open up discussions around it, as well as seeking professional help for them and yourself.)

I get so many emails from partners asking me to help their loved ones change their drinking habits and I always reply by saying, 'I can't help anyone unless they personally reach out to me for help. They have to *want* my help for me to be able to help them.'

I can remember lying in bed reading quotes to Gus while he was trying to sleep about the various cancers he was making himself vulnerable to and the depression he may develop as a result of his drinking. Preaching? Much? Gosh, I cringe when I read this.

It was all coming from a good place, but I realise now how bloody hypocritical it sounded when only a couple of months earlier I'd been begging him to grab me a bottle of wine from the bottle shop on his way home from work! What I know now with experience and hindsight is that we are more likely to positively impact our partners through our actions and not our words.

LET'S REFLECT

Take a moment to reflect on your relationship and how focused around alcohol it is/has been by answering the following questions.

1. How much has alcohol featured in your relationship since you met?

2. Do you have any shared hobbies/activities that you regularly engage in that don't include alcohol?

3. How resistant is your partner to you not drinking? (If you haven't directly asked them this question, what do you think their thoughts are?)

4. How connected do you feel to your partner when you aren't drinking alcohol?

Six transition changes

Reflecting honestly on the questions above can offer you some insight as to how difficult removing alcohol will be on your relationship. This in turn can help you consider how smoothly these next steps might go.

In order to navigate any changes in our relationships as seamlessly as possible, we need to work through six important transitions.

1. Share openly and honestly where you're at and why you're making this change (but that you don't expect them to change if they don't want to).

2. Navigate, discuss and mutually agree upon the boundaries that you want to put in place regarding drinking behaviours (theirs), socialising (both) and expectations around these.

3. Check in on them through the process.

4. Communicate your feelings through the transition to prevent disconnection and to navigate sober sex (more on this later).

5. Create a shared ritual of connection.

6. Create new shared interests and goals.

When we have a blueprint of 'how' to navigate the changes sobriety raises in a relationship, it makes it so much easier. Gus and I didn't and we definitely learnt the hard way! I hope me sharing this makes it easier for you! Yes, it takes commitment and work – but surely that's worth it for your mutual happiness and future in the long run?

SHARE OPENLY AND HONESTLY

While it's important that we don't preach or expect our partners to come on this journey with us, it is also important to communicate openly and honestly about why you're doing this and what you might need from them along the way.

Letting your partner in on your journey is crucial to ensure you stay connected, feel supported and have a safe place to each share how you're feeling while this big change and transition takes place.

You need to have an open and honest conversation about *why* you are doing this, the detrimental impact alcohol has been having on you (which you may not have honestly shared before), and ask them for their support, whatever that looks like for you. If you haven't yet done this, consider how you might do so by completing this sentence below.

I am making this decision to take a break from alcohol because _____ and it's really important I have your support so that _____. I know this might bring about a shift in how we spend time together and I would love for us to consider some activities that keep us connected while I am navigating this change.

Some partners, if they don't have a dysfunctional relationship with alcohol themselves and are an 'every now and then' drinker, may not understand your need for complete abstinence.

I've lost count of the number of times clients have told me that their partner wants them to stop drinking so much but doesn't want them to stop altogether and can't understand why they can't just enjoy a glass or two over dinner every now and then.

If this resonates with you, ask your partner to read the section where we discuss drinking in 'moderation' and why it doesn't work for so many people in Chapter 1. Hopefully, this will help them understand why it isn't a case of 'just having one' and they will need to support you if you choose to completely remove alcohol. They can't have it both ways: picking and choosing when it suits them for you to drink.

Initially, I wasn't honest with Gus. I didn't share the impact alcohol was having on my mental wellbeing, my sleep, my anxiety, the constant swirling thoughts in my head, always thinking about when I would drink next or how much I could have or whatever new rule I was creating. I didn't tell him about the self-loathing, the self-disgust that I experienced most mornings, or the fact that often, once I'd dropped the kids at school, I would crawl back into bed and play Candy Crush most of the day because I had little motivation or interest for anything else. I didn't tell him that I felt like I was slowly rotting inside. Instead, I pretended I didn't have any kind of problem with alcohol but that I just wanted to 'lose some weight and increase my energy'.

Part of this was (strangely) about feeling ashamed that I couldn't 'handle my booze' anymore after years of using my alcohol stamina as a badge of honour with little negative consequence. I felt a bit like I was letting Gus down if I admitted it wasn't working for me anymore when it had been such a big part of our lives (and many of our wonderful memories were booze-fuelled events I still look back on fondly). I thought I was weak and that he would be disappointed with me for not drinking with him.

Now, if only I had spoken to him in more detail, I would have realised he wanted to support me. I just didn't give him the opportunity and I simply kept putting on the act that everything was 'fine' when inside I was, in fact, crumbling into a million little pieces. (I think most of us in this situation would be in the line-up for the 'I'm Fine' best actor Oscar of the year.) With any of our significant relationships (not just romantic partners but our friends and family members, too) it's important we open up and talk about how we are truly feeling and our real reasons for taking this break from alcohol, as it can save so much heartache further on in our journey. It also creates a deeper connection in the relationship because we can feel much more supported and understood.

> **Talk with your partner and loved ones – be open and honest. Share the impact that alcohol has been having and ask for their support.**

NAVIGATE AND DISCUSS BOUNDARIES

Establishing your boundaries together is the missing piece to preventing arguments and hurt feelings. Start by considering what boundaries are important to you when it comes to how and when your partner drinks around you.

Perhaps your boundary is that they don't drink at home around you, they keep their booze in a separate fridge so you don't have to see it every day, that they don't buy you alcohol to try and coerce you into drinking with them (yes, this has happened to several of my clients after they've declared they are taking a break from booze, and then Friday night their partner arrives home from work with a bottle of their favourite bubbles).

Doing this upfront work together is vital to avoid difficult conversations or situations later on. It's about working out the actions that will allow you to feel more supported. I've made some suggestions for you on the next page as to what I've seen work, but you may like to consider what would apply in your own relationship. It's important this is communicated in the way it's intended – with positivity and as a constructive way of working through potential barriers or obstacles.

LET'S REFLECT

When discussing possible boundaries to help you in your decision to remove alcohol, what might work for you? Here are some examples.

1. Alcohol in the home – can it be stored in a different fridge or area so you don't have to see it? Can you ask your partner not to drink at home in front of you?

2. Not nagging if your partner wants to go out for a few drinks and comes home a bit drunk, but also establishing that you don't want to be left sitting alone at home all the time. What compromise can be made here?

3. When you go out together socialising, you don't always want to stay until 2 a.m. and watch them and everyone else get smashed and then be the Uber driver home. Let them know what time you are likely to want to leave, explain they don't have to come with you (if this works for you) and they can get a lift or a taxi home later if they want to stay.

Your boundaries are:

1. _____

2. _____

3. _____

CHECKING IN: HOW IS IT FOR YOU?

Something we often forget to do when we take a break from or remove alcohol is ask our partners the simple but often very revealing question: 'How is it for you now that I'm not drinking?' Remember – it's not all about you! They will be experiencing a significant period of readjustment, too.

We can get so wrapped up in our own sobriety, in doing 'the work', in healing, growing and connecting with new sober friends who we feel understand us more, that it's really easy to forget our decision does impact our partner too. While that's not something to feel guilty about, it is something to acknowledge.

When we go on this journey of removing alcohol, it's inevitable that other changes will happen, as we have already discussed. We start becoming curious about what triggers us and why. We open our minds to new ideas, new ways of spending time, finding new friends, discovering new experiences. We begin to want more because we believe we deserve more. (Hell yes, we do!) Our confidence grows, our energy increases, our hopes and dreams get bigger. We are no longer happy to settle for a 'less than' life and want to move from simply existing to truly living. And while this is amazing and incredible and exciting and new, it can be scary as hell for our partners who are watching it unfold with fear, uncertainty and insecurity. In many cases, they've lost their drinking buddy and this can feel confusing and scary. And they may not know how to express their feelings about it, to you or anyone.

One of my clients was talking to me in one of our sessions about how her partner seemed withdrawn, disinterested and unavailable to her. I put it to her: 'Have you asked your partner how it is for them, watching from the sidelines as you go on this journey of deep transformation and change?'

She hadn't and so agreed to do this. The following week she shared the outcome. 'We went for a walk and I asked him, as you suggested, how he was going with my decision to stop drinking. He replied, "It's scary as hell. I'm watching you do this work on yourself, and I can see how much happier you are, but I'm scared. I'm scared if this continues that I won't be enough for you anymore and you will leave me."' I smiled, as I had expected this response. I hear it time and time again. It's scary for our partners when we make a major change, especially if it's one that they aren't making alongside us. In many cases, they want to support us, but they don't know how.

If we want to prevent disharmony and conflict in our relationship as we embark on this journey, it's important we allow our partners space to share.

Talking openly and sharing your experiences along the way, as well as asking them how it is for them, ensures you stay connected and your partner doesn't have to feel threatened. By asking them that question we are sending a message that they matter, too, and we want to know how they feel. We give them space and permission to share.

EXERCISE: CHECK IN REGULARLY

Take time to check in with your partner throughout this transition phase with questions that show them you care, you are interested in their thoughts and you want to listen. This allows for open, honest and authentic conversations that only serve to deepen and strengthen your relationship.

Examples of questions you can ask are:

1. 'Are you noticing any changes since I went alcohol-free that you would like to discuss?'

2. 'Is there anything you're worried about that you'd like to discuss?'

3. 'I know it's a big change and I want to make sure you can talk about this. What's this like for you?'

UNDERSTANDING AND COMMUNICATING OUR NEEDS

Remember in Chapter 5 we talked about our needs in a variety of contexts, including our relationships? One of the most important needs we have is for belonging, safety and connection in our relationships. When we remove alcohol, this is a really important time for us to begin to understand and communicate our needs.

If you were having a crappy day, feeling lonely, disappointed and disconnected, would you say to your partner when they walked through the door, 'I feel really bad today, can I have a hug?'

So many women I've asked this question respond with, 'No way!' Would you?

Why do we find it so hard to ask for what we need? Firstly, it stems from the fact that we don't often know what we need and secondly, we feel vulnerable asking for that need to be met. The thought of 'What if they say no?' might go through our head or 'What if they think I'm weak or I'm failing?' Displaying vulnerability means we feel exposed.

Revealing our vulnerability means taking a risk with no guarantee of the outcome (as described by research professor at the University of Houston, podcast host and author Brené Brown, known for her work on vulnerability and shame). But when we do, it also means we create a more authentic, deeper connection.

I remember on one of our newly ritualised evening walks, I shared with Gus how a flippant comment he'd made the previous evening had hurt and upset me. I explained that while I knew that probably hadn't been his intention, nevertheless that was the outcome and I asked if in the future, he could use a less attacking tone when he wanted to discuss this prickly topic. We talked about why it had upset me so badly, how he could have said it in a less attacking style, and we both ended the conversation feeling understood, heard and validated. It was a huge step forward for us as a couple and me as an individual.

Starting sentences with 'I feel' or 'I need' instead of using statements that start with 'You', which places the emphasis on the other person, makes a huge difference. I encourage you to begin to ask yourself the question: 'What do I need right now?' when it comes to your relationship, followed by: 'How can I express that need in a healthy manner?'

You might recognise you feel disconnected to your partner, so you ask them to go for a walk and share your feelings which might cause you to both work out how to create time to connect more. It might be you feel you would like more physical intimacy so you can ask your partner if this is the case for them, too. It might be that you don't feel appreciated for all you do so you ask to have a weekly 'I appreciate' meeting where you share what you have appreciated about the other person over the last week. (Yep – we did this and boy, did it work!) Communication is vital and it's the key to staying connected while navigating this normal but nonetheless disconcerting change in your relationship.

Consider what you might like to say. Here is an example for you.

'I'm feeling _____ *and it helps me feel close to you when I share how I'm feeling. I'd love for you to share your feelings too. I'm recognising I need more* _____ *in our relationship and this will help us stay connected*

during this transitional time. I would love to spend time with you this weekend and wouldn't it be great to try _____ as a new activity together.'

LET'S TALK SOBER SEX

We can't talk about learning to express our needs in a relationship and navigating the changing dynamics without also talking about sex.

As we age, many of us find we become less confident in the bedroom – put it down to bodies that have grown babies, constant comparison to what we see portrayed in social media, porn and advertising as to what a woman 'should' look like, and then throw in changing hormones, reduced libido and no Dutch courage to relax us and get us in the mood, and it's no wonder sex, even with our partners, can feel awkward and intimidating.

I conducted a poll in one of the alcohol-free challenges I ran, in which I asked the women, most aged between 40–60, when they last had sex with their partner sober. Most couldn't remember.

The respondents revealed it was common for them to use alcohol before sex to distract themselves from feeling shy, to give them more confidence between the sheets and to help them relax. However, the issue is that while alcohol is a depressant, meaning it does relax us, it also numbs us, so we don't fully experience all the pleasurable physical sensations of sex. They had been doing this for so long that they couldn't recall when they'd last had sex without drinking first. It can be daunting. But sex without alcohol is nearly always better! I get so many emails from women sharing how much their experience of sex has improved when they aren't numbing themselves with alcohol, and how much more intense and satisfying it is. In one of my alcohol-free challenges I interviewed Sober Influencer Jodi Clarke about her experience of becoming sober. I asked her, 'What has been the most surprising thing about your alcohol-free life?' Her response? 'How much better orgasms are!' And she is so right! Studies show that some women under the influence of alcohol have a decreased intensity of orgasm.

Let's understand why. According to research in the National Library of Medicine, alcohol use causes testosterone to drop. Lowered testosterone in men leads to fatigue, lowered libido, decreased sperm production, shrinking testicles and erectile dysfunction. In women, it can lead to hair loss, fatigue, poor sleep, weight gain, depression, anxiety, reduced libido and an inability to have orgasms!

When I've run polls in my groups about the benefits of sobriety, so many women of all ages and from all over the globe back up what Jodi said: 'The sex is so much better!' For most of us, we've been using alcohol as a gateway to sex for so long that we don't know how much better the sex can be without it.

What so many of my clients find is that once they get over their initial discomfort or awkwardness around sober sex, the actual sex is infinitely better.

But how do we get in the mood without our trusty ethanol depressant?

In an interview I did with sex therapist Jacqueline Hellyer back in 2021, she made a really valid comment. 'We are happy to talk about where we want to go on holiday and what our favourite food is but so many of us struggle to shares our likes and desires in the bedroom.' So true! Isn't it more important to understand and share our sexual fantasies than whether we want steak or fish for dinner? And yet so few of us do. Not to mention that as we age, our preferences change. What we liked aged twenty is probably completely different to what we like aged 50. Especially in the bedroom! Communication is key here.

As Jacqueline says, 'Mature sex takes its time, appreciates all aspects of the experience, doesn't set out to hit "goals", just enjoys the experience as it unfolds.' I highly recommend Jacqueline's website and articles for some brilliant and practical information and tools on improving your sex life at any stage of your relationship.

Remember:

- Talk more and communicate your desires with your partner, as well as sharing if you feel nervous or shy.

- Spend time on foreplay which doesn't have to be sexual – connecting, hand holding, hugs and time spent together is all foreplay.

- Go slow and enjoy the moment. Any sexual encounter doesn't have to end in intercourse.

- Great sex starts with how you communicate outside of the bedroom. Showing interest, and feeling appreciated, heard and important in your partner's world are the most effective ways to improve your sex life. It's hard to have incredible sex when you don't feel seen, understood or loved. Start with those areas first and notice how this increases your desire to become more intimate.

LET'S REFLECT

Take a moment to consider the following:

☐ How often have you had sober sex with your partner?

☐ Do you feel daunted at the prospect? (It's totally normal if you do.)

☐ Can you find a time to talk to your partner about this often delicate topic and share any of your insecurities, needs and desires?

☐ Prioritising time for sex is important, as is taking time to get in the mood. Can you set aside time for date nights, a trip away or morning lie-ins?

REDISCOVER A RITUAL OF CONNECTION

In the past, the main way Gus and I connected was over a shared alcoholic drink to mark the end of the day, decompress after work and have a chat together. He'd get home from work and grab a beer, a signal to me to grab the wine I'd had chilling in the fridge, and we'd head out to the garden for a quick catch-up. Sometimes this involved a sneaky fag behind the washing line while the kids watched *Peppa Pig* and then we would head back inside, not only caught up on each other's news and feeling seen and heard by the other, but also perhaps just a little elated after a brief moment of rebellion behind the washing line against our adult responsibilities.

After I stopped drinking, we stopped doing this. I began to feel 'different' and this had created a divide between us. I felt like I was on this path of self-discovery and healing and he wasn't. This left us feeling distant from each other and, I will admit, I felt fearful and unsure about our future together.

Discussion between us seemed to focus only on the logistical planning of our kids' after-school activities, along with delegating weekly household chores. We'd stopped talking about our lives, our dreams, our hopes and our goals. We'd pretty much stopped talking at all and it felt like we'd lost any common ground.

I do believe that every marriage goes through periods like this. We don't have to remove alcohol to experience something similar as the increased responsibilities of kids, mortgages, careers and household chores puts a stop to a lot of the hedonistic and spontaneous social lives we had before. But removing alcohol really does shine a spotlight on any communication breakdown because you don't have that shared drinking time together.

So it wasn't really a surprise when we soon found ourselves sitting in a couples' therapy room, nervously hopeful but also filled with resentment and frustration towards each other, about to encounter the wonderful German couples' therapist named Wilhelm.

'I can see the biggest problem here,' Wilhelm said. 'You have no ritual of connection. When you removed the alcohol and stopped sharing those evening drinks together at the end of the day to talk, connect and listen, you stopped connecting altogether.' And he was right.

When I quit drinking, we had stopped the evening check-in and connection, that moment of giving our undivided attention to each other, no matter how brief. We didn't even realise we'd stopped, it just kind of happened, and we had no idea how important that ritual of connection had been in making us both feel acknowledged and seen by the other.

When Wilhelm pointed this out, it made so much sense. And while our new evening ritual of sitting down for a cup of tea together, or heading out for a dog walk after dinner didn't feel quite as rebellious, it helped save our marriage.

It's important to create new rituals of connection, which could include:

- a shared sporting activity together (pickleball, tennis, squash, gym bike rides, walks, hikes, running)
- morning coffee or breakfast together before the day starts

- evening walks to talk about your day and show interest in each other

- a moment when you both return from work and check in with each other without phones or other distractions, giving each other your undivided attention, even if just for five minutes

- having 'what went well' chats over dinner or as you get into bed, sharing with each other what's gone well for you that day

- having 'I appreciate you' meetings – a connection point once or twice a week to share something you appreciate the other has done that week

- date nights that aren't just sitting in a restaurant staring at each other trying to think of something to say; try going to comedy shows, theatre, day trips to local places of interest, cooking classes, language lessons.

Once we create these rituals of connection and moments to check in with each other, we begin to feel more aligned, seen and heard (something we all need so much). When we feel that way, we feel closer to our partner. And when we begin to feel seen, heard and connected, we then feel able to start talking about the future together and what that might look like, without alcohol.

LET'S REFLECT

Take a moment to consider what new rituals of connection might work in your life. Write down three that you could suggest to your partner and pick the one you both want to start with.

1. _____

2. _____

3. _____

SOBRIETY IS ...

'Discovering myself each day, finding freedom and continuously raising my life to new levels.'

JADE

'Meeting myself as an adult for the first time.'

BELLA

'Being in control of my life and my future! Sobriety for me is a massive feeling of contentment.'

BRIDIE

CREATE NEW SHARED INTERESTS AND GOALS

So few of us take time to evaluate and audit our lives as we age. We outgrow hairstyles, fashion and music (well, some of us – I still love rave music but now I listen to it when I'm running, not off my head on the dance floor!) so it makes sense we outgrow the activities we do in our spare time, especially those we do together, which for Gus and I had been partying and drinking.

But we get lazy and this is true in many marriages – irrelevant of whether we quit booze. We stop making the effort and if there's one thing I know in all my years of marriage, it's that when we take our foot off the gas and become complacent, cracks will quickly begin to show, especially if we've been using booze for connection and then we remove it.

Initially, new activities might feel quite 'lame' – no evening dog walk together can give the same dopamine hit as a bottle of wine – but revamping your rituals and discovering new shared interests together is essential and can be lots of fun!

When I think about Gus hiding under the blanket in a yoga class like a scared rabbit as all the flexy lululemon women downward-dogged and happy-babied around us, I actually burst out laughing! Nope, yoga definitely wasn't his thing. But it warmed my heart that he gave it a go. And similarly, my lack of coordination on the tennis court and actually throwing the racquet and storming off when he served one Roger Federer–style ball too many makes me cringe now! But we tried and we had a go at doing new things.

What works for us now? Walking and hiking in the bush, cooking classes, family board games, fishing (well me reading, him fishing but both loving time together on the ocean), British crime dramas, running, travel, comedy shows, live music, zip-lining, telling stories round the fire, bike rides and exploring new places.

Don't worry if you don't find mutual interests the first time you try. Just be open to continuing to experiment and trying new things together to discover what works for you both in *your* relationship.

In his book *The Seven Principles for Making Marriage Work*, author and Professor of Psychology John Gottman says, 'Marriage isn't just about raising kids, splitting chores and making love. It can also have a spiritual dimension that has to do with creating an inner life together ... an appreciation for your roles and goals that link you and that lead you to understand who you are as a family.'

Creating a vision board around your shared goals and dreams is a brilliant exercise I encourage you to complete together. Ask yourselves where you'd like to be in five years, what personal dreams and goals you have, and what joint ones you share. When we did this exercise, we talked about retirement, where we wanted to live, the holiday home we wanted to buy, the travel we wanted to do, the hobbies we wanted to have time for. It bought up conversation topics that we'd never discussed before and helped us feel closer and more aligned.

Sometimes doing this exercise can be a little confronting and brings up some difficult questions. Maybe you value different things, especially if you aren't drinking but your partner is. Maybe you have very different goals or visions for the future. Yes, this can be unsettling but isn't it better to have these discussions than to avoid them and remain in a marriage where you are not truly aligned? And if you realise that your goals and values aren't currently aligned, it doesn't mean the marriage is over. It just means a lot more communication has to happen. While Gus and I are aligned in some things, we absolutely aren't in others and knowing this is really helpful, too. We can give each other space and time to explore the things we separately love while prioritising time together for the activities and interests we jointly enjoy. If things get a bit stuck when having these big conversations, then I recommend couples' therapy. It saved our marriage and it might just save yours, too.

LET'S REFLECT

Some questions for you to answer together while you are creating your shared vision board.

☐ Where do you see yourself living a year from now, five years from now, ten years from now?

☐ Will you move house or stay where you are?

- ☐ Do you have any grand travel plans?

- ☐ Do you have any individual goals you haven't shared with each other before?

- ☐ What's on your bucket list? (If you haven't created a bucket list this is such a fun activity to do – 30 things you want to do before you're 80.)

- ☐ What age do you want to retire and what does retirement look like for you?

- ☐ What financial savings goals do you have between now and then?

- ☐ What health goals do you both have?

- ☐ Are there any career goals you want to achieve before you retire?

- ☐ Do you see yourselves staying close to your children or other family and will this influence where you live?

- ☐ What don't you want your retirement to look like? (This question offers some real insights.)

Sometimes it just doesn't work out

Do some marriages or relationships end when one partner (or both) quits booze? Yes. But I don't believe this is actually *because* we are no longer drinking. I believe it's because there is nowhere to hide anymore from the issues in the marriage. When we remove alcohol, we shine a big spotlight on what isn't working.

When we are unhappy in our marriage, alcohol becomes a crutch. It distracts us from the pain and misery that we don't want to acknowledge if our marriage is crumbling and it allows us to not have to deal with difficult decisions. We simply avoid facing what's in front of us by drinking our sadness away.

When we remove alcohol, any niggling doubts we had about our relationship can sometimes become glaringly obvious. And with the clarity and inner confidence that comes with sobriety, we have the impetus to do something about it. But it's important not to act too quickly or have a knee-jerk reaction. Any period of change requires time to adjust.

I've seen couples who thought they would never make it become happier and more connected than they've ever been, after a period of adjustment. I've also seen clients do a lot of work on themselves, and on their marriage, and reach the conclusion that separation is the right path. This has led to them becoming their most authentic and happiest selves. There is no right or wrong.

Any big decision needs to be carefully considered, and working with a couples' therapist, even to navigate a separation, can be incredibly beneficial, especially when there are children involved.

All the single ladies

So what if you are sober and single? Or find yourself single at some point? How on earth do you meet new partners, alcohol-free? I've worked with many clients who are looking for their life partner and, for perhaps the first time, doing this completely alcohol-free. Eeeeek!

An increasingly common way of meeting potential partners is through dating apps. However, according to the team at Resurgence Behavioral Health, 'over 70 per cent of people on top dating apps drink, and many will propose a first date that involves drinking alcohol over a sober date, believing that booze will calm their nerves and break the ice.'

For many single, newly sober people, this can feel somewhat overwhelming and disheartening. However, there are ways to navigate your way through this, if dating apps are your thing.

The first step is to decide whether you want to include your sobriety on your online dating profile. The second decision is whether you want your prospective partner to also be sober or if you are happy to meet someone who does drink. It's not about being a preacher and shouting from the rooftops that everyone must quit drinking, as we've previously discussed, but it is about deciding your own personal boundaries and clarifying what would be an issue for you with a potential new partner's drinking.

There are several dating apps entering the market that are specific to non-drinkers, such as Loosid (USA) and the website Single and Sober (for UK, Australia, USA and Canada). The apps Hinge and Bumble have specific features you can use to indicate if and how often you drink. This allows you to discover how much another person drinks before deciding if you want to date them.

Also, do look at some of the brilliant sober meet-up groups that host events across the globe to meet like-minded individuals for sober fun, friendships and romance (more info at the back of this book). This can be a less daunting way of meeting others on the same path.

Only you can decide what your boundaries are on the topic of a potential partner's drinking and what you are comfortable with. I have some clients who couldn't consider dating anyone who drinks, whereas others are happy if it's someone who is a 'take it or leave it' drinker but not a regular or heavy drinker.

Sober dating also prevents you making impaired decisions when it comes to sex, and being less likely to regret any behaviours we may have participated in when drunk.

Some ideas for sober first dates include meeting for a walk (always easier to talk when walking!), going to a comedy show, having coffee or lunch, or seeing live music.

One of my clients, who was single and dating sober, met a guy who she had an incredible physical connection with but realised very quickly that they just weren't aligned in so many areas of their lives. Due to her newfound clarity she was able to make the considered decision not to continue the relationship. She said: 'Old drinking me would have carried on for months and brushed aside the fact we had such different values, outlooks and beliefs, simply to enjoy the sex, but new sober me knows she wants more than that – a truly deep and authentic connection that ticks *all* the boxes, not just one.' Through ending that relationship, she made room for a wonderful man to come into her life who has ticked every single box! There's nowhere to hide when we aren't drinking, which can be a huge benefit when dating sober.

Remember, there are many benefits to dating sober, as it allows you to really get to know someone without the altering impacts of alcohol on their (and your) personality.

Your sober partner pact

As I come to the end of this chapter, I've hopefully given you lots to think about when it comes to your own relationship and your partner's experience of your sobriety.

The biggest point to consider is that we can't remove alcohol and expect everything in our relationship to remain the same. We have to look at what we are adding *in* when we've taken alcohol *out* of our relationship, and we have to expect a period of readjustment.

Change can be hard and overwhelming. Don't make any hasty decisions during this period of adjustment, and consider couples' therapy if it's available to you.

Your relationship *will* change, and in many cases, for the better after a period of readjustment. Just be as prepared as you can be for the transition that lies ahead.

SOBER ACTION STEPS

☐ Talk openly about your reasons for removing alcohol.

☐ Set boundaries that you're both comfortable with about where alcohol features in your relationship.

☐ Keep checking in with your partner to ask how it is for them.

☐ Check in with your own needs and communicate them to your partner – they aren't mind-readers!

☐ Create small rituals of connection that will work in your unique relationship, such as:

- evening walks

- discussing what went well

- 'I appreciate' meetings

- date nights.

☐ Discuss shared activities, goals and visions for your future life together.

JOANNE

I gave up drinking alcohol while I was in the middle of (what I thought was) a healthy relationship. We were in the first year so we were still in the relatively early stages when sex was particularly exciting (or so I thought).

When I stopped drinking, my boyfriend also stopped to be supportive, and so we embarked on sober sex together. But oh my, the pressure I placed on myself! *'I have to be sexy, I have to make it happen.'* Plus, all the unwelcome body confidence issues rose to the surface. But to my surprise, with my new sober mindset and confidence, it felt good. It was enjoyable (at the time) and I felt proud that I could do it. I was owning this sobriety thing and my life was improving. However, with the alcohol removed, the red flags that I had been conveniently ignoring were becoming more ominous. Our connection was dwindling and the sex was becoming less enjoyable.

Fast forward two years, I finally removed myself from what transpired to be a narcissistic relationship which left me hurt, betrayed and angry. But the sober me was able to feel the feelings, process what had happened and heal.

Meanwhile, the prospect of sober dating was a bit daunting, as I'd only ever gone on drinking dates. Through my inner sober work, I realised that I felt very differently about myself.

I felt precious, worth protecting, even vulnerable. I didn't want to let just anybody in. I appeased myself with the idea that I could go on lunchtime dates, or breakfast dates, and that the kind of man I wanted to meet wouldn't need to have a boozy date to enjoy himself.

However, it triggered insecurities: What were these men going to think of me? Were they going to judge me? Would they think I was boring? I also found myself thinking of the flip-side – what sober guys are even out there that I would want to date? How do I find them? Can you meet sober guys on dating apps? Do people post that they are sober?

With all these questions spinning around in my head, I decided to park dating for a while. I was busy living a full and glorious sober life; I decided I didn't even need to date.

And then I met a beautiful man. A 'glass of wine with a meal occasionally' type of man. A man that enjoyed his life, was ambitious, had great energy and didn't need alcohol to be on the menu for a great night out, or to spend the day doing something nice.

The attraction was strong and mutual. We couldn't keep our hands off each other. The sex was mind-blowingly intentional. It was intense and it felt wildly empowering. When sex isn't fuelled by the sloppy mess that accompanies alcohol, you realise just how beautifully intimate it can be. You want to feel every touch, you want to taste every moment and you definitely want to remember it!

Over the next eight beautiful months our sexual relationship grew. We took our time. We learned how to give each other pleasure. It was never rushed. It was open, we communicated, we stopped for breaks, we shared what we liked and we tried new things that neither of us had done before. I felt safe. I felt looked after. Without doubt I know that if alcohol had played a part, we would not have had this experience. I wouldn't be able to remember a lot of it and I certainly wouldn't have wanted to write about it. And those muggy-headed morning hangover wake-ups and the feeling of dread of what we'd done the night before?

We didn't have any of those either.

CHAPTER 7
SOCIALISING SOBER
Yes, you can do it!

'Let's catch up when you're drinking again,' my friend flippantly called over her shoulder one day at the school gates, as we were both dashing off to get our kids to after-school activities. I'd just overheard her talking to another friend about a catch-up they had planned the following evening, which I hadn't been invited to presumably because I wasn't drinking. While it was not intentional, that comment hurt me deeply.

'But what if I don't ever drink again,' I thought, 'does that mean we can never hang out?' With that came a surge of spiraling, negative thoughts that projected the future, sober me as lonely, sad and miserable. I wonder if you've had this experience too?

Do thoughts like these prevent you from making the changes that you actually want to make in your life but fear of loneliness and losing friendships holds you back? I get it. I've been there, too.

Navigating friendships when we make changes in our lives, especially changes that involve some kind of personal growth, can be tricky, and sometimes more so than having to deal with changes in our romantic lives!

As women, we are often incredibly loyal. We may have friendships we've fostered for decades, built on history, shared memories, having kids at the same time. We pride ourselves on the longevity of these friendships and sometimes place more emphasis on the length of time we've been friends than whether we still have anything in common.

My friendships have changed and evolved in the years I've been on my sober journey. Female friendships have always been important to me. In many ways growing up, they became more important than my family in terms of whose opinion and love I needed and craved most. There was nothing I wouldn't do for my friends. From my own research I know now that if we grow up in a family where we don't always feel seen or understood (the case for so many), we turn to our friends more than ever. As I've aged, I have continued to invest as much time, energy and love into my friendships but I also don't have as much time and energy to give while juggling children, work and running the home, so my friendship group has become smaller. But with that shrinkage in size, the depth and quality of the friendships have increased. I think sobriety has played a part in this, too. I'm just not interested in surface-level chat anymore. I'm not interested in gossip, comparison or competitiveness. I want friendships where I can be my true, authentic self. Where I don't have to put on an 'act' and adapt myself to what I think people want me to be. Who has energy for that?! I care less about what people who don't matter think of me. I care more about being authentic, having honest conversations (which can cover a wide range of topics from abortion rights to bowel movements to sex to shades of red lipstick!), and feeling seen and supported for who I truly am.

I know quickly when I meet someone if they are 'my' person. My body tells me. If I feel like 'me' in their presence I know they are a keeper. If I feel a tightness in my tummy or chest, I know I'm not in the presence of someone who makes me feel like 'me'. Of course, a huge part of this journey has involved having to discover what the true, authentic 'me' feels like, which has been a bumpy roller-coaster, but I'm learning more about myself every day. Do you know when you feel most like yourself? Who are you with? What are you doing? It's this gentle self-inquiry that supports us on this journey. Yes, there have been friendships I've let slide because I realised they were based around alcohol and not much else, or recognised our values, beliefs and goals were so vastly different I struggled to find a middle ground. And it's truly okay to walk away from relationships that don't serve us anymore. As we will soon discuss, not everyone in our life is meant to be there forever.

Just because it's always been like that, doesn't mean it has to stay like that

So often I hear women say to me: 'We don't have anything to talk about when we aren't drinking, but we've been friends for 30 years so I can't just end it.' We might feel vulnerable, scared and uncomfortable when we come to this point and it can cause us to question our decision to be alcohol-free. We know we are better without it but sometimes we feel such a deep sense of loyalty to others (I know women who have gone back to drinking to keep their friends happy), or fear that we might never make new friends so we return to drinking even though we know it doesn't work for us.

But if we navigate this shift in our friendships with openness and effort to keep the connection going, a deeper and more authentic connection can be created in a way you never expect. We can also make room for new, incredible friendships to form that are relevant to this stage in our lives.

There comes a time when we need to prioritise ourselves in these friendships instead of carrying on doing something we no longer want to do simply to make others happy.

PASSENGERS ON THE TRAIN

Something that helped me so much with this complex and often highly emotional stage in my sobriety was the passage, 'Angels on a Train' by John A Passaro. The passage describes life as being like a train ride, with different people getting on and off our train at different stops, and that it is normal and to be expected that not everyone will be there for the whole ride.

This is my favourite part from Passaro's passage:

Be very wary of people sneaking on at certain stops when things are going well and acting like they have been there for the whole ride.

For they will be the first to depart.

There will be ones who secretly try to get off the ride and there will be those that very publicly will jump off.

Don't pay any heed to the defectors.

Just know where and how people get off is more of a reflection on them, than it is on you.

Be blessed for the ones who get on at the worst stops when everyone else is departing.

For they are special.

Always hold them, dear, to your heart.

For they are the important ones.

Like a train that stops at several stations, I have found there are several stages we transition through in our friendships when we are navigating changes in our lives (such as sobriety!) that also impact those around us. Some friendships last the distance, and some don't and that's okay. As Oprah Winfrey says: 'Surround yourself with only people who are going to lift you higher', and I couldn't agree more.

You may also have heard the famous quote: 'People come into your life for a reason, a season or a lifetime.' Not everyone is meant to be there forever.

Let's look a bit more deeply at four stages you may move through as you navigate changing friendships and learn to socialise sober.

STAGE 1: RESISTANCE

The first stage is resistance. If we have a solid friendship group that has involved frequent drinking together, there is nearly always going to be resistance from others when we quit. It's important to recognise that while we often interpret this resistance to be unsupportive and, at times, really hurtful, often that is not the case.

As with our partners, our friends are often scared that our decision to take a break from alcohol will mean that we won't connect with them anymore. They fear losing us as a friend. They fear not having anything in common with us. They fear being judged for their own drinking. And they fear us changing and 'leaving them behind'.

While these emotions are all valid in this situation, the issue is that many people don't have the vocabulary or insight to recognise what is really going on for them or, if they do, they don't know how to articulate it. Their communication can feel coercive ('Oh go on, you can just have one, don't be so boring'), unsupportive ('I don't know why you're doing this, you don't *need* to take a break from alcohol') or sometimes downright cruel ('If you quit drinking we won't be able to be friends anymore').

We *can* transition through this resistance stage and still sustain incredible, deep and authentic friendships while also making room for *new* friendships to come into our lives.

From one passenger to another

I want to make a confession here. I was the absolute *worst* friend in the past when those closest to me said they weren't drinking.

I was enraged if a friend wasn't drinking at an event that I had already planned in my mind would be a fantastic night of us getting drunk together. I felt rejected, disappointed and let down. I remember one year, ahead of my annual birthday girls' trip to Rottnest Island (a day that started with drinking at 11 a.m. on the ferry over and continued with all-day drinking at the beach, followed by an evening dinner that few of us remembered), my friend Jen said she hadn't been feeling well and might not drink at Rottnest. I was horrified. I couldn't understand it. I felt like she was letting me down. I'm ashamed to write this now, but my response was that she may as well not bother coming if she wasn't going to drink.

With hindsight and some years of sobriety now under my belt, I can see that the reason I responded like this was due to my beliefs around alcohol and the fact they were truly ingrained with the idea that we couldn't have fun unless alcohol was involved. In my experience, it's mostly people who don't have any issues with alcohol who don't have issues with us quitting, and it's the people who do have issues who feel threatened and judged by our decision to quit.

It's often the case that the only people who have a problem with us not drinking are those who have a problem with drinking.

Something I didn't do, and which I wish I had done either early in my sobriety or in the lead-up to quitting, was to talk openly and honestly with my closest friends about the impact alcohol had been having on my mental and physical health.

If I had, I do believe I would have saved myself a lot of pain and hurt feelings. As with so many of my clients, no one truly knew the impact alcohol was having on me. Yes, everyone knew I was a big drinker and loved a party but if anything, this was something to be applauded and was never seen as negative. I didn't share the crippling anxiety I would often experience, the sleepless nights, the fear that my life was passing me by and I wasn't even playing a part in it, that I was simply sitting on the sidelines like a bystander with no say in what direction it took. I didn't share the feelings of shame, hopelessness and fear that often riddled me and I didn't share that some mornings I couldn't even look at myself in the mirror because I despised the woman staring back. No, I kept it all inside.

If I had opened up more, especially at the start, the conversations would have been different, I'm sure. I usually just said something along the lines of: 'I'm trying to lose weight; I've been going too hard and need a little reset detox.'. Why do we do this? Generally, it's because we feel ashamed that our drinking has got to the point where we need to do something about it, and this is only exacerbated by our cultural stigmas around alcohol addiction.

Perhaps we also feel we are letting others down if we stop drinking. It's the irony of alcohol – we are shamed for drinking too much and shamed for not drinking enough or for developing a problem with what is one of the most addictive substances in the world. And then there's guilt, because we feel it's our responsibility to make sure everyone around us is happy, and they won't like it if we quit booze.

I can't tell you the number of women I've worked with who have loved everything about sobriety but have gone back to drinking because they felt bad that their friends didn't enjoy them not drinking. As with our partners, opening up, being honest and sharing our feelings is how we can navigate this stage. It helps also to set appropriate boundaries around who we share the truth with and who gets our standard response. 'I'm taking a break and feeling *so good* for it, I'm going to keep going' is a comment that few can respond negatively to.

STAGE 2: ACCEPTANCE

Once we reach the stage of acceptance, our friends realise that we aren't just doing a five-day juicing detox that will end in a celebratory piss-up at the local wine bar as per previous breaks from alcohol. (I once celebrated in true style: at the end of a 21-day sober stint I had a colonic irrigation to 'cleanse' my internals before meeting all my mates at the pub, gleefully excited that I would get pissed much quicker seeing as my insides had just been cleared!) When our friends realise our sobriety is going to be long-term, one of two things generally happen. They accept and carry on, adapting to this change in our friendship, or they begin to distance themselves.

And this can be the time that some friendships do fall away. In some cases, this happens naturally and easily and although we may notice, we don't necessarily mourn the end of that particular friendship.

In other cases, it can be more painful and hard to accept. Perhaps it's a friendship we would have liked to keep going but the other person pulls away. There is only so much we can do here. In some instances, it's about evaluating if this is a friendship we want to fight to maintain (by reaching out and talking openly to your friend) or whether it's a friendship that we realise isn't based on much more than drinking, even if it's one we've had for ten, fifteen or twenty years. I do believe that in some cases friendships are meant to end to allow us to grow in the way we need and also to make room for new friendships to come into our life. So many incredible women have come into my life since I removed alcohol, and other friendships have slipped away.

In his book *Necessary Endings*, Dr Henry Cloud writes: 'If we cannot see endings in a positive light and execute them well, the "better" will never come either in business or our personal lives'. He argues that our personal and professional lives can only improve to the degree that we can see endings as a necessary step to something 'better'. And this is certainly true in this scenario of some friendships ending that no longer feel aligned or serve us anymore. As an aside, I think this is also true in general with regards to ending our relationship with alcohol. If we see it as a negative ending, we will mourn its loss. If we see it as a positive ending, we will celebrate all that this new lifestyle decision offers us.

For those friendships that we know are worth investing in and prioritising while we move through this clunky, awkward stage of sobriety, there are three things to keep in mind.

1. **Make sure you keep conversations open and honest**.
   Share with your friend that their friendship and support means the world to you. Check in how it is for them with you not drinking (like we do with our partners). Understand that they will also be managing complex emotions while we go through this change. Keep the lines of communication open and honest.

2. **Prioritise time together that involves new activities**.
   Don't just meet in wine bars and watch them get sloshed while you sip your Diet Coke and pretend you're having a great time. Meet for walks, activities, coffee, live events or plan things to do together that you both enjoy.

   I have created new ways of socialising with my friends which include early morning sunrise walks (my fave!), Sunday morning yoga and coffee, monthly comedy nights, evening runs, ice baths, saunas, sober raving and theatre visits. It's taken intention and planning but it's been so important for me to maintain connection with the friends I love outside of back-garden wines and weekend piss-ups.

3. **Know (and set) your own boundaries, particularly early on**.
   In early sobriety, going to big events like concerts, weddings, birthdays and holidays all felt way too hard and overwhelming to navigate without a drink in hand. Nowadays I look forward to them even more because I know I will remember them, and not feel like shite the next day. (And yes, I do get on that dance floor and shake my booty while completely sober! It has taken time to get to that point but slowly my sober confidence has grown!)

   Take baby steps at first when navigating bigger events. Take alcohol-free drinks if you can – that doesn't just limit you to Coca-Cola! There are plenty of alcohol-free options for beer, wine and even gin. They have saved me so many times. More and more places are starting to stock alcohol-free drinks as sales of these are rising – yay! I've included a list of my favourites in the resources section at the back of this book.

Plan what you will say if someone asks why you're not drinking or what you would like to drink. Know that you don't have to over-explain especially to people you don't know well, and be clear on when you'll leave the event and how. I also find it really helps to have something great planned for the following morning so you don't feel like you're missing out if you do leave early once everyone else is drunk. Some ideas might be an early morning yoga class or run, brekkie with a friend or the family, or a sunrise beach walk where you can reflect on how great you feel.

Celebrate socialising sober: be present and have authentic connections with everyone you meet, then drive home whenever you want, feeling energised and proud (because you haven't made a dick of yourself).

LET'S REFLECT

1. Have there been friendships in your life that resonate with you now as having been for a season? Do you remember a particular friend who you were close to at school that, at the time, you couldn't even consider a life without, but you haven't spoken to in years?

2. Where in your life are you recognising a friendship may not go the distance if you're no longer drinking? How do you feel about that? What would you miss about that person? Is the friendship one you want to fight for? Recognise if a friendship has turned toxic and no longer supports you.

   A useful tool is to ask yourself, 'How do I feel when I'm with that person?' and 'How do I feel after I've spent time with that person?' It's a clear clue as to whether we are showing up as our true, natural authentic self and if we can still connect and have fun with this person without alcohol.

3. Consider the people in your life who you really want to prioritise. Think about who you might want to talk to about your sobriety and ask for their support. Go back to the exercise in Chapter 5 where we talked about our needs. What are your needs in a friendship and are they being met?

STAGE 3: A PEOPLE TREE

After we've realised that some of our friendships will naturally fall away and identified those we truly want to invest in and work at, it can be helpful to consider who the people are that influence us the most. You may have heard the saying 'you are the average of the five people you spend most of your time with'. Have you ever actually sat down to consider this in detail?

In neuroscientist and author Dr Tara Swart's book, *The Source*, she has an exercise called 'the people tree' where you list the five people who have the greatest influence on you and then describe the character traits of each. This helps us to consider the energy, influence and mindsets of the people who influence us the most. We can also consider the role alcohol plays in their lives to be able to understand how removing alcohol from ours might impact that relationship. Dr Swart describes our connections to these five people as crucial and states that the quality of the connections 'has a huge influence on our thinking, mood and behaviour'.

Once we have drawn up our own people tree, we can consider who brings out the best in us, who inspires us, challenges us, motivates us to be the best version of ourselves. We can also see who tries to keep us in a small box, unchanging and staying as we always have been, or constantly drains us of our energy and stays stuck in negative thinking patterns, never open to change. This can be a clue to consider where changes in friendships may be needed in order to make way for new friends who inspire us and celebrate our journey of change. It's often the case that these new friends are on the journey of change themselves. Achieving success in areas we want to change comes from exposing ourselves to new ways, new thoughts, new ideas and sometimes new people who push us out of our old thinking patterns and beliefs. If we stay in our old echo chamber for months or years on end with people who aren't open to change, it's unlikely we will find the growth or change we seek. Stepping out of our echo chamber is a crucial part of the process.

It's also important to note that the journey of transition might mean some people fall away and then come back to us. This has certainly been the case for me. At first it felt like the friendship may not survive but through time, patience and acceptance, I found that some people reached out to me a year or so later and said things like, 'I admire you so much. I need help with my own drinking, how do I quit?' or 'I want what you have.' Never underestimate how much you are impacting others without realising it. Some friends need time to adapt and that's okay, too.

EXERCISE: CREATE YOUR OWN PEOPLE TREE!

Consider the five people you spend the majority of time with or who have the biggest influence on you.

1. _____

2. _____

3. _____

4. _____

5. _____

Next add five words to describe each person and their traits (no one has to see this so you can be honest).

Consider how you feel when you're with each of these people and after you've spent time with them. Do they leave you feeling upbeat, inspired, positive and truly seen? Or do you leave feeling drained, exhausted, misunderstood or perhaps not seen at all because they often dominate the conversation?

Once you have reflected on these five people, think about who you need to insert boundaries with and who you want to spend more time with. By setting boundaries you can free up time and energy to invest in new friendships that may be more aligned to this new stage of your life.

SOCIALISING SOBER

'I thought I would feel awkward in social situations where everyone is drinking but I feel more confident and calmer.'

ZOE

'I can now stand tall and proud after a party. '

JO-ANNE

'I can have clear, coherent and intelligent conversations that I won't cringe about the following day.'

BEC

STAGE 4: ADD NEW

The women I've found I love to connect with most in my sobriety (outside my core group of girlfriends), are ex-drinkers like me. Put a group of ex-piss-head women in a room together who've 'done the work' on themselves and be ready for the best conversations of your life! These women are some of the most interesting, real, authentic and inspiring women I've had the privilege to meet ... and they are everywhere! The connections, energy and atmosphere these women generate lift to a completely different vibration than if they were all drinking. Once when I hosted a sober event in Sydney, the people working at the venue said they had never experienced such an uplifting, positive vibe and couldn't believe everyone was sober!

I have made some incredible connections since quitting booze and a couple of these have been formed 100 per cent online. The online sober community is an amazing place full of support, encouragement and honesty – one of the biggest pluses of social media in my opinion! Take, for example, my friend Fleur. We met on Instagram in 2020. We both commented on a post by a sober influencer asking where people were from. Fleur commented she was from the UK, living in Australia. I replied, 'Me too.' We took our chat out of the thread and into DMs, asking how long we had each been sober (I was just over a year and Fleur was a few months ahead of me). We shared a love of sobriety, running, rave music, collagen supplements and fashion. There has rarely been a week gone by since early 2020 where we haven't had some kind of contact and, in April 2023, I flew to Sydney where we met for the first time in real life! Amid squeals of excitement and happiness we spent 48 hours together, barely stopping to catch a breath.

Fleur has been a constant for me through so many transitions in my life over my sober years and it proved to me you don't have to be 'in person' friends to create a deep, authentic connection. Sobriety is such a common ground for creating new friendships. The resource section at the back of this book has recommendations for sober meet-up groups. And if you haven't already, do join my Facebook community 'The Women's Wellbeing Collective' for a supportive, warm and welcoming community of women on a path to self-growth and discovery. The theme for the group is: 'Sit with women committed to personal growth, the conversation is different.' Making space for new friendships to form and meeting like-minded women with similar interests has brought me and so many others incredible joy. It is one of the key benefits of my sober life – there is nothing quite like the sober community for welcoming you with open arms and warm hugs.

LET'S REFLECT

If you feel ready to add new authentic friendships into your life, let's consider how you can do this.

Join sober meet-up groups. There are so many all over the world! The sober community is the most warm and welcoming community and there are sober events and parties popping up everywhere from Perth to London to New York and Sydney. See the Resources section for some ideas. And if you're in Perth join my Facebook group 'Perth Sober Socials' for monthly events I host around town.

Think about hobbies and interests (more on this in the next chapter) that you would like to explore. It's a quick-win way to meet like-minded people as you are both doing an activity you have interest in. I have clients who have made friends through running groups, paddle- boarding groups, cycling groups, walking groups, dancing groups, choir and pottery groups.

Complete this sentence:

Meeting new like-minded people is important to me because _____. I am going to do this by _____ and my first step is to _____.

What you gain,
not what you lose

Johann Hari says in his famous TEDx talk: 'The opposite of addiction is not sobriety. The opposite of addiction is connection', and I truly believe this to be the case. So many of my clients drink because of loneliness. Some have found that they have pushed people away in order to stay at home drinking and want to hide this from others. They don't want to have to 'control' their drinking which they feel they have to do when in public.

Others are drinking because they are generally lonely and want to numb this feeling. We have to remember that humans are built for connection. When we consider our hierarchy of needs, outside of food, water and shelter, love and belonging are our two most important. Hari also describes loneliness and lack of human connection as key reasons for the development of depression, and this has been supported by research.

I see time and time again in my coaching that loneliness and lack of connection are key reasons for women drinking. The fact is, we can have a wide circle of friends but still feel lonely. Because if we don't feel seen, understood and appreciated as our whole, authentic self, it's lonely as hell. If we have to 'act' in some way in a friendship, it's probably not for us. And that's okay. Learning who and what makes us feel good in ourselves is part of this journey of self-discovery. It doesn't happen overnight but gradually, subtly, and as we begin to peel back the layers, we begin to recognise the people in our lives who make us feel most like ourselves.

Being intentional in stepping out of our comfort zone to meet new people is important to ensure we are still *adding* to our lives when we take alcohol *out*.

While navigating these changes in both our romantic and platonic relationships does take work, it is important to note that it's through this work that we create deeper and more authentic connections. I do believe that we get out what we put in and I apply this logic to every area of my life.

As you've already heard me say, it doesn't all just land in our lap exactly as we want it, we have to work at it. Want great, authentic friendships and a deep and supportive marriage? Both take work, commitment and intention.

Creating deep and authentic relationships, without the mask of alcohol, takes courage, commitment, vulnerability and effort. When we put that in, we get so much out.

SOBER ACTION STEPS

- [ ] Communicate your feelings.
- [ ] Explore new ways to hang out with your friends that don't involve alcohol.
- [ ] Consider who you may not have a deep friendship with outside of drinking and know that it's okay to let that particular friendship go.
- [ ] Be intentional about creating new connections through local groups and events.
- [ ] Lean into the online sober community, which is warm and welcoming.
- [ ] Accept that change means we are growing and, while there can be resistance on both sides, this is normal. It takes time for all parties to adjust to change. Be patient.
- [ ] Take steps to build new connections in different areas of your life.

FLEUR

At sixteen I started smoking and drinking every Saturday night. I always wanted to drink and smoke. Drinking took away any worries, and insecurities just disappeared in that drunken haze. Drinking and having a blast on Saturday night with my friends became my hobby. Even back then I had no off switch. I would drink until there was nothing left and was often unable to remember the end of a night.

This pattern repeated itself throughout my 20s and 30s. But when I had my son in my late 30s my drinking changed. I wasn't working and I would use wine as a reward for getting through the day at home. I found being at home quite boring and my nightly couple of glasses of wine perked the day up a bit.

When I went back to work my drinking changed again, back to more binge-drinking on the weekend. The one thing that was constant was how I used alcohol. If I was bored, I would drink; if I was sad, I would drink; if there was an event or a party, I would completely write myself off. The effects of a big night would take me days to recover from.

My drinking had impacted the way I thought about myself. I was overweight, moody, irritated and had a persistent feeling that I could do so much more with my life. There were a few people I knew who were fit and healthy and seemed to have a hugely fulfilled life. This was something I really wanted but felt there was no way I was going to be able to get as I spent too much time either drinking or nursing a hangover. I was trying so hard to put on a big, smiley face it was becoming exhausting.

The big turning point for me was when I was 44. My friend died very quickly of cancer. It really scared me. She was very healthy and rarely drank. This made me think: if she could die from cancer what on earth would happen to me? I was terrified that the life I was leading was paving the way for disease. Let's face it, it certainly wasn't helping prevent disease.

This was the exact moment I decided it was time for change, even though I wasn't sure what that looked like. I started to run with a friend to help lose some of the weight I had always battled against. We ran the Mother's Day classic race and the feeling of doing something fun and healthy with like-minded people ignited a fire inside of me. I loved it! Then we started training for a half marathon, and I wondered what it would be like to run without a hangover. So that week I decided that I would give up alcohol for the next 60 days before the race.

As the race got closer, I had decided that I never wanted to drink again. I had finally found something that I was enjoying more than drinking. Meeting friends to run with on Sunday morning gave me a reason to not drink Saturday night. Getting up early to run on the trails was giving me everything booze had promised but didn't deliver. I had this brand-new social life that was centred around being happy and healthy.

When I removed alcohol from my life, I knew I would need to fill the huge gap it would leave. I added in running and the domino effect of a healthy life took over. I cleaned up my diet and no longer craved the high-calorie fatty foods I consumed every weekend during and after drinking. One of my favourite things in the world is to see the sunrise and I try to do this as much as I can. It means I am welcoming another day that I can fill full of thoughts and activities that make me the best version of myself.

Since I have given up drinking, I have completed so many trail-running races that I have lost count. I run at least three marathons a year. Last year I set myself a challenge to sign up for my first 100-kilometre ultra marathon. Taking part in this race is one of the most incredible experiences I have ever had in my life. When I crossed the finish line, I was the proudest person in the world. I had just done something that I had dreamed of; I was finally the woman I wanted to be. My new dream is to complete a 160-kilometre race in the mountains. My dreams are getting big!

CHAPTER 8

WHAT'S YOUR FUN PLAN?

What to add *in* that brings more joy and interest to your life

'I may just pop in to show my face but I won't stay long, there's no point if I can't have a drink.' How many times have you caught yourself saying something like this as you knock back the chance to be social when you're doing something that feels very anti-social, like abstaining from alcohol?

I remember saying words to this effect to my friend back in 2018, when we were planning an upcoming birthday party for one of our girlfriends. I was on yet another 'diet', partaking in an eight-week exercise and no-booze challenge at my local gym to try and lose some of the weight I'd been gaining with my excessive drinking and late-night cheese-and-crackers binges.

At that time my mindset was that if I couldn't drink, there was no real point in attending any social occasions. Or if I felt obliged to go, it would be a fleeting hello and a quick goodbye so I could retreat to what I considered my boring sober existence, checking my calendar to see how many days to go until I could have actual fun again. I thought any period without alcohol meant a 'less than' life: something to be endured, crossed off, days counted down to simply 'do the time'. Boy, did I have it all wrong.

For years we've been fed the story that alcohol plus socialising equals fun and that sober plus socialising equals boring. Has this been your mindset, too? For so many of the women I work with, this is the part that keeps them going back to booze time and time again. Our belief that we *need* alcohol to have fun is just so deep-seated we fully believe that we *can't* have fun without alcohol.

One of my favourite quotes of all time is from the founder of the Ford Motor Company Henry Ford: 'Whether you think you can or you think you can't – you're right.' The story we tell ourselves is what becomes our truth. In this case, the story is, 'I can't have fun without alcohol.'

This is where I call bullshit!

What we need to do is challenge this belief. You could start by asking: 'What does having fun actually mean or involve for me?' Creating a life we love, without alcohol, means examining why we think we need it to enjoy life. Part of this is discovering what *actually* lights us up in an authentic, present state and doesn't require a mind-altering substance that simply dumbs down our brain to make boring things seem more interesting. I mean, let's just honestly reflect on that. What kind of life do we really have if we can't enjoy ourselves without alcohol? If we need alcohol to make things seem more interesting, then are we really interested in those things?

As author Mark Manson puts it: 'If you need to drink to enjoy a person or thing, you don't actually enjoy that person or thing.' BOOM! So true, right?

Let's have a look at what those changes might be. Later in the chapter we will look at *how* we make them.

Honestly, if we need alcohol to love our lives,
we need to change our lives!

What even is fun?

Let's start by defining what 'fun' is. The Oxford Dictionary describes fun as 'enjoyment, amusement, or light-hearted pleasure'. For me, it's something that has no purpose other than for your own enjoyment. Something you do that is only for *you*.

I wonder what this is for you? What do you do regularly that is purely for your own enjoyment and pleasure? (Outside of drinking, of course.) Not for your kids, not for your partner and not to make other people happy. Perhaps you're like I was and your answer is actually not much at all.

We've already established in Chapter 5 that it's essential we set boundaries and prioritise ourselves to create a life we love and one where we no longer want or even need alcohol. If you're stuck wondering what else to do with your freshly discovered time and energy, this is what we need to explore further now. And this is where doing the work can be life-changing.

Even if you're a social person like me who loves being around other people, 'fun' doesn't have to always mean being with others. Sometimes I find fun in being in my PJs on a Friday night at 6.30 p.m., happily curled up on the sofa with my daughter watching a movie, eating popcorn and debating whether we love Patrick Swayze more in *Point Break* or *Dirty Dancing* (*Dirty Dancing* every time, right?).

Fun isn't about living the 'perfect' Instagram lifestyle. It's not defined by how great our lives appear on social media or by what restaurants and bars we go to. Fun is about being with the people we love and/or doing the things we love that bring us deep, personal joy in that moment. And surely deep, authentic connection with the people we love is more fun than boozy nights, not remembering anything that happened, then waking up filled with shame, regret and anxiety?

When we redefine fun for what it actually is – things that we do for our own joy, interest and happiness – so much opens up and we start to realise there are so many ways to have fun outside of simply drinking.

So many of the women I speak to in sober communities drank or are drinking because they are bored. If you recognise boredom as a trigger for you, it's time to explore what you need to add in for fun, joy, pleasure and interest so you no longer need to drink to make your life less boring. In our modern world we are so distracted by smart phones, social media, gaming and sometimes alcohol, we have become afraid of boredom. We don't want to let it into our lives, even for a moment. But in fact, boredom is where magic can happen. Dr Anna Lembke, the author of *Dopamine Nation*, says:

> Boredom is not just boredom. It can also be terrifying. It forces us to come face to face with bigger questions of meaning and purpose. But

boredom is also an opportunity for discovery and invention. It creates the space necessary for a new thought to form, without which we're endlessly reacting to stimuli around us, rather than allowing ourselves to be within our lived experience.

In boredom we can actually discover who we are and what we love because we aren't being distracted from ourselves.

I find it's when we go through transitional stages in our lives that boredom can really rear its head. For example, after we have kids and are home a lot more, or when our kids move out or get their driver's licence and suddenly we are not needed to drive them around or organise their lives. Or we might be working in a job that is all-consuming and leaves us so exhausted that all we have the will to do is drink each evening to forget about it. It's often after busy periods or seasons of life we find that, now that we have more time, we don't know what to do with it. It can feel confronting and uncomfortable and so we drink. Recognising this is key. We then have to look for and create opportunities for things we find fun and enjoyable, not simply wait for them to come to us ('cause we'll be waiting a long time!).

When we begin to change our beliefs around what fun is and start adding in the activities and experiences that light us up, we begin to create more joy and fulfilment in our lives.

So first, how about we do a quick audit on where things stand for you.

LET'S REFLECT

1. What do you do currently that is just for you that doesn't involve alcohol (and please only list exercise if it's something you actually love as opposed to something you feel you should do)?

2. Over the last five years, how many experiences can you reflect on that have lit up your soul, left you with a warm sense of gratitude and love, and haven't included alcohol?

3. What hobbies or activities did you enjoy doing at any stage of your life which have slipped away but which you would love to pick up again if there were no limits around time, money or opportunity?

SHORT-TERM PLEASURE VERSUS LONG-TERM HAPPINESS

It's important we also discuss the difference between activities that evoke short-term pleasure and those that bring us real authentic joy and happiness as, in my mind, they are quite different. Short-term pleasure activities, something we also call 'instant gratification', affect the dopamine reward centre of the brain, causing it to really light up when we engage in them. And what we now know is that there are companies out there working round the clock to create and sell us products and experiences that do just that so we keep going back for more. Think excessive shopping (particularly online), sugar and processed food, social media, alcohol, gaming or gambling. Many of these are promoted incessantly and are available to us instantly. We buy the product or engage in the activity, and once the initial buzz has worn off (the dopamine high), we are left wanting more. We might even feel a little flat afterwards (this is going into a dopamine trough).

On the other hand, authentic joy and happiness are often completely free and are activated through our serotonin (contented happiness) neuro-transmitter pathway rather than our dopamine pathway. When we experience activities that create a release of serotonin (or oxytocin, the human bonding neurotransmitter) we feel more contented and fulfilled than the quick high we might receive from the dopamine-inducing pleasure activities. Consider the enjoyment you get from experiencing connection with a loved one, having a beautiful meal with your family, or hiking to the top of a mountain and pausing to experience the awe of the magnificent world we live in. It's essential to pay attention to where we turn for pleasure, joy and happiness, and identify if it's something that's being 'sold' to us or something we truly, authentically love. Remember our glimmers and dopamine tickles we discussed in Chapter 3? One of the greatest gifts of sobriety has been this innate sense of contentment within myself that I just didn't have when I was drinking. I now often find myself having moments of being overwhelmed with gratitude and love for my life, our natural world and much more. This never happened when I was drinking.

> To create a life we love, we have to discover the activities
> and experiences that bring us true, authentic joy and
> challenge our existing beliefs about alcohol.

What do you believe?

In Chapter 2 we discussed our first introduction to alcohol, and also what we observed of our parents' drinking.

As I've shared with you, the message I picked up at a young age was that the way you had fun as an adult was by drinking with your friends. That was when I saw my parents laugh the most, when they seemed happiest and when my little brain must have joined the dots to create this belief. Of course, I didn't recognise this was happening, but psychologists tell us that we create most of our unconscious core beliefs about life, the universe and ourselves before the age of seven.

I have spent a lot of time with clients unpicking those core beliefs and disputing them, helping them see that just because we formed a belief about something aged seven doesn't make it true, and doesn't mean it is how we have to live life and make decisions as an adult aged 47. We are excellent at turning opinions into facts. But we do need to be careful of doing that as we can end up missing out on so much. When we create the belief: 'I need alcohol to have fun' for example, we immediately go into any experience that doesn't involve alcohol believing it won't be fun. Once we turn this belief around to: 'I have fun when I'm with the people I love doing things I love', the old belief immediately gets quashed.

EXERCISE: UNPACK YOUR BELIEFS

Before we go further, I encourage you to write down your beliefs around alcohol and then explore them. The following questions can help:

☐ What was the message you received early on in life about alcohol?

☐ What beliefs about alcohol did you grow up with? How was it modelled to you?

☐ How did that integrate with your own experience when you started drinking?

Now let's try some turnaround statements:

- [ ] 'I can't have fun without alcohol' can become 'I have fun when I'm doing things I love with the people I love'.

- [ ] 'Sober socialising is boring' can become 'Going to events where everyone's sole intent is to get as drunk as possible isn't how I enjoy spending my time. I would much rather do something else, such as _____.'

- [ ] 'I need alcohol at parties to have confidence as I'm too shy without it' can become 'I'm naturally an introvert and big parties aren't really my thing. I much prefer spending time in smaller groups where I can be my most authentic self'.

For so many of us, we've stopped doing anything for our own pleasure outside of drinking so now we get to explore doing other things for fun!

Who are you now?

I know we've talked a lot about stress and setting boundaries, and how many of us are too busy, too overwhelmed or feel too guilty taking time for ourselves that we continue putting up with a mediocre life for fear of rocking the boat.

But it's essential in this commitment to our new fulfilling and happy sober life that we discover who we are right now and what we love at this age and stage and season of our lives.

Whether that's as new parents, parents of teens managing their changing hormones while often simultaneously navigating our own hormonal changes (what an absolutely shitshow that can be!), being consumed with work or being empty nesters, we need to make a commitment to peel back the layers and uncover what truly lights us up and what we enjoy doing. It's a process of self-discovery, one that reaps so many rewards if we take the time to do it, experiment and be open to trying new things and saying yes to doing things differently.

Because let me ask you this: have you changed from the person you were when you first started drinking? Do you still enjoy watching the same TV shows, reading the same type of books and wearing the same clothes? My guess is no – you've evolved, matured and have different tastes now.

So why haven't we considered that what we might like to do for fun in this season of our life has probably also changed?

I believe the answer to this is that we have simply never paused to reflect on this question (or any of the other larger life questions that I've posed throughout this book) because we've rarely (if ever) been prompted to do so. Wouldn't it be amazing if at every major milestone in our lives, every turn of the decade, instead of getting smashed and vomiting into a plant pot (yep, been there, done that) we paused to evaluate our life, what was working and what wasn't, what we enjoyed and what we didn't, who we loved hanging out with and who we've naturally outgrown, so we had information and facts to know what we should and could change for the decade ahead. Imagine what a life we'd have if we did that!

This is what it takes to create a life you love without booze. It takes challenging your old beliefs around alcohol, reflecting on what is and isn't working in your life, setting boundaries so you have more time, and then beginning the joyful and revealing experiment of working out what you do actually love to do for fun as the incredible woman you are today. And if you don't know right now, that's okay (and very normal!). We can work it out.

And as with everything else we've been covering in this book, it takes *actively deciding* to make the effort to do this self-discovery work, to get to know yourself as the woman you are today, pledging that you will lean inward and listen to what you really think, and let what you really love shine through, and not be distracted and manipulated by big companies constantly selling quick-fix products as the solution to your boredom and disillusionment.

**It's time to work out what you love to do
for fun as the woman you are today!**

TIME FOR ME

'My life has opened up. I have replaced alcohol with gardening, art and furniture restoration. And I have a part-time job that I love.'

NESS

'It's been amazing to be able to have just as much fun – if not more fun – without drinking!'

HAILEY

'I have expanded levels of confidence and SO MUCH TIME! I had no idea how much time was involved in planning, thinking about, and recovering from the drinking.'

JO

Redefining 'fun'

It should be clear from the start that fun means doing something with the sole purpose of it being for your own happiness and joy. This doesn't have to mean getting dressed up, going out with a huge group of friends and getting absolutely trollied. In fact, I would argue that this is anything *but* fun for most people. Especially for those of you who have discovered in sobriety that you are actually quite shy, introverted or hate big groups (which is why you were drinking in the first place).

Fun is when we spend time doing anything we authentically love, whether that's dancing, studying, gardening, reading, horse riding, singing or learning. We just have to start discovering what that is for each and every one of us, something that many of us have forgotten along the way while parenting, adulting and looking after everyone else.

A fun experiment that starts now!

As we begin to explore the activities and experiences that we can add *in* to our lives, there are three traits we need to have on board: saying yes, being curious and being open.

We are all different. On this journey of self-discovery and experimentation, we don't have to go along with societal norms (often created by big conglomerates with billions of dollars in their pockets trying to convince us we have a 'less than' life if we're not consuming their product).

1. SAY YES TO DIFFERENT

On our quest for sober fun, happiness and joy we need to start doing things *differently*. We can't do everything we used to do with a drink in hand and still expect to get the same enjoyment out of it. The likelihood is we won't.

A client emailed me last week to ask: 'Sarah, will I ever have fun again? I spent all Sunday afternoon at a beer-tasting festival with my friends and I found it so boring. I couldn't wait to leave. I don't want to drink but I don't want to feel bored every time I socialise with my friends.' I smiled as I typed my response, which was this: 'I can't think of anything worse than spending hours at a beer-tasting festival when I'm not tasting beer! Of course you can have fun when you quit booze, but you have to say yes to doing things differently – changing how you spend your time and being open to trying new activities instead of instantly dismissing them to do the things you always used to do, but are now doing without alcohol.' What could you start saying yes to that is different to how you spent your time before? (Some ideas on this below.)

2. BE CURIOUS

When our curiosity is piqued it's a clue that we are interested in something. And spending time doing things we are interested in is fun and ensures we experience more joy. Most of us live on complete autopilot, never noticing what piques our interest, and so we never listen to the clues we are being offered every day. Starting to be aware what piques your curiosity is key. We can also be curious about the times we experience jealousy, as this is another great clue to what we might be interested in doing/having/achieving. We've been taught that jealousy is a shameful emotion to be kept hidden but what if we became curious about our jealousy? I believe it has a lot to teach us when we choose to explore it, as it's showing us something we want which we might not currently have. And there is absolutely nothing wrong with wanting something!

3. EXPERIMENT AND BE OPEN

Deciding to take the step of experimentation is key here. We need to experiment to discover what we love doing. If we've been doing nothing for ourselves other than drink for the last three decades, we can't know immediately how we want to spend our time. And me telling you what I've discovered is fun may be your idea of hell, so that doesn't work either. Instead, you need to commit to going on a journey of individual trial and error which, in itself, is all part of the fun process. It's a win-win situation but we have to be open to trying and not simply dismissing ideas based on old thoughts, beliefs and experiences. See this as an adventure. As Helen

Keller said: 'Life is either a daring adventure or nothing at all.' We have to remember that this part of the journey takes effort, too.

My own experiment to discover what I loved doing for fun once I'd ditched the booze has been enlightening. It includes activities Drinking Sarah would never have considered fun. In fact, she would have turned up her nose in disgust! But hey – this is what I mean about appreciating the fact we evolve and change as people and giving ourselves *full permission* to do so.

For me it's a mix of early morning hikes watching the sunrise, ice baths, breath work, an afternoon fishing with my family, dinner with a girlfriend trying new restaurants, jigsaws (what the hell? Drinking Sarah never would have done a jigsaw!) comedy shows, bike rides, zip-lining, live music, degustation menus, Pictionary, reading, studying, listening to podcasts about the brain and neuroscience (yep, turns out I'm a geek at heart and just didn't know it!), sunset walks on the beach, attending workshops on topics like nervous system regulation or creating the perfect flavour of tea, sober dancing (especially in the kitchen at breakfast time), hot yoga and so much more. When I did the renowned VIA character strengths survey, which is a free scientific-based character assessment tool, my number-one top strength was love of learning, and so now I understand why when I'm learning something I'm in my happy place. (You may wish to do the survey, too. You can find it at viacharacter.org)

When we move away from our old belief that fun has to mean socialising, we can start to see that fun is *anything* we do for our own pleasure. Then the whole world starts to open up. It's incredible!

EXERCISE: EXPERIMENTING WITH FUN

Listed opposite are some of the activities that my clients have engaged in once they quit booze which you might like to try. They are so different! Some may really jump out at you, and some may not. If you notice an instant reaction of 'OMG. No way!' come up as you read through the list, challenge that reaction. Why? Is it that you think you 'can't' do it or you won't be good enough, or do you feel too intimidated to start? Remember, everyone has to start somewhere.

Put a tick next to the ones you might like to try.

ACTIVITY	WANT TO TRY?	HOW I FEEL ABOUT TRYING IT
Joining a hiking or walking group		
Joining a local theatre group (acting, set design, helping with costumes)		
Singing lessons or joining a choir		
Learning a musical instrument		
Dancing classes or group (e.g. tap, ballet, jazz, Zumba)		
Fitness classes or group		
Volunteering at an animal shelter, food bank or women's refuge		
Cooking classes		
Interior design classes		
Aromatherapy course to learn about essential oils		
Creative writing classes		
Going back to uni/Tafe to study something that interests you		
Adopting and training guide dogs		
Learning a card game		
Landscape design, gardening, growing your own vegetables, horticulture classes		
Photography classes		
Knitting, crochet, sewing		
Pottery or art classes		

I encourage you to pick one activity that you would like to try in the coming week.

Complete this sentence:

Something I would love to try (or return to as an activity I enjoyed when I was younger) is _____. Adding this into my life will make me feel _____. It may also open up the possibility of meeting new, like-minded friends. This is important to me because _____. I am going to do this by the following date:_____.

Positive emotions

As we talked about earlier, discovering new ways to experience more happiness and positivity means we create a life which gives us joy and, subsequently, we feel less of a need to drink. With that in mind, I want to introduce you to the ten core positive emotions as listed by Professor of Psychology Barbara Fredrickson in her book *Positivity*. When we realise that adding more positivity to our lives doesn't have to involve huge life changes but small, simple tweaks and steps, we feel more empowered with the knowledge we *can* create a more positive mindset. Adding positivity can take nothing more than being more present and savouring the experiences in our life, instead of always rushing past them. This comes back to what my 80-year-old self often whispers to me: 'Slow down Sarah, enjoy the journey without always rushing to the destination.'

This quote by author and Associate Professor at Hardin-Simmons University in Texas Melissa Madeson really appeals to me:

> When individuals can explore, savour and integrate positive emotions into daily life … it improves habitual thinking and acting. Positive emotions can undo the harmful effects of negative emotions and promote resilience.'

I have listed Fredrickson's ten positive emotions and my view on them in the following pages because when we take every step we can to evoke these positive emotions in our lives, we feel happier. Our brain is naturally wired for survival, so it's always on the look-out for threat and danger. To overcome this natural tendency we can teach ourselves to savour positive emotions.

These ten positive emotions may just help you in your journey of exploring what makes *you* happy and deciding what you want to add into your life for your own simple happiness hits.

As you read through this list, I encourage you to think about where these emotions feature in your life currently or what steps you could take to add them in.

1. SERENITY

Think for a moment about what serenity means to you. When did you last experience this emotion? If you're anything like me, it's probably not a word that enters your vocabulary much. For me, serenity is a sense of absolute calm and quiet. It's the absence of pressure and rush. It's a moment to pause, breathe, connect within and simply 'be'. I experience this most when I'm either in the yoga studio or the breathwork studio, or I'm lying on my bed listening to a yoga nidra. I also experience serenity when bush walking and all I can hear is birdsong.

Slowly but surely, I begin to slow down, my shoulders drop and my breathing deepens. And in that moment, I feel truly content because there is nowhere else I need to be, other than just in that moment. Allowing myself these small moments of serenity throughout the day enables me to face the more demanding and high-pressure tasks with more ease and calm. Notice when and where you feel this sense of serenity. Make it a priority to spend more time in this place. If serenity is not featuring in your life at all right now, consider what you could add in to support you here.

I can add more serenity into my life by _____.

2. PRIDE

I always try to check in with myself at the end of each day and ask myself the simple question: 'What am I proud of today?' Pride is such an important emotion when it comes to feeling more positive and happier in our lives.

Some days the list is long. 'I'm proud of the way I handled that tricky situation with my kids' teacher; I'm proud of not flying off the handle when the kids broke my favourite coffee mug playing water ping-pong with it;

I'm proud that I finished that really hard book I loved but found super challenging; I'm proud that I went for a run even when I wanted to stay in bed another half hour because it meant I started the day feeling energised and positive.'

Sometimes my list isn't like that at all. Sometimes it's simply, 'I'm proud I didn't pick up a drink today.' Regardless, there will always be something to experience pride for, even if it's small in the grand scheme of things – it's still something. Make sure you find it.

I commit to ending each day by completing the sentence: Three things I'm proud of today are _____.

3. INTEREST

Finding ways to do things that genuinely interest you completely redefines what fun actually is. If you'd told me a few years ago that I would classify a fun weekend as driving to a scout camp in the middle of the Australian bush to spend 48 hours with a bunch of strangers learning breathwork and cold water therapy, and ending it with a five-minute ice bath, I would have laughed in your face (while lighting a fag and pouring a wine – obvs!). But I loved every single minute of this experience because I was learning about things that interest me.

As discussed, the fact that I love learning is something I've realised in my adult, sober life. And now having time to spend learning about things that really interest me is a gift and a joy. In his book *Deep Work*, author and Professor of Computer Science Cal Newport talks about the fact that the human brain actually loves and needs to be stimulated and challenged. But being stimulated and challenged is not always the same as being busy. We can spend a day being really, really busy but not actually doing anything that stimulates or challenges our minds. We then get home and feel we deserve to switch off and numb out after a busy day, so we may stare at the TV with a drink in hand or endlessly scroll on our phones but, in fact, our brain is crying out for stimulation. Newport says:

If you give your mind something meaningful to do throughout all your waking hours, you'll end the day more fulfilled, and begin the next one more relaxed than if you instead allow your mind to bathe for hours in semi-conscious and unstructured web surfing.

Time and time again I see in sobriety many of us developing this incessant thirst for knowledge and stimulation from topics that really interest us, because we finally have the energy, clarity and motivation to act on our desires. I often ask in my group coaching program, 'If you could go back to university now and study anything at all, what would it be?' The responses are always amazing. Criminology, art history, psychology, film making, photography, architecture. The list is endless.

Now I'm not suggesting we can all ditch our jobs and income and go back to uni, but I am suggesting that many of us, when gently probed, do have an idea of what we might like to learn more about. And not because a teacher told us or a boss told us but because it's genuinely what interests us now, at the age we currently are. Listening to podcasts, reading or doing an evening class on the topic can be a great starting point. 'Find what interests you and do more of that' is my motto here.

Topics I am interested in learning more about are _____.
I am going to explore this by _____.

4. GRATITUDE

Having a genuine gratitude practice can be life-changing. Truly appreciating what we *do* have instead of what we *don't* have can completely change our mindset about life and create so much more positivity. Our subconscious brain is more susceptible to new thoughts in the first twenty minutes after waking which is why so many coaching and mindset gurus will encourage you to do your gratitude practice, affirmations and visualisations at the start of the day. It can be done in any form you choose – written, thinking, saying out loud. Some evidence suggests there is more benefit from writing but in all honesty, simply starting a gratitude practice in any form will benefit you.

Starting the day with what I appreciate about my life has seen me through some tough times. There is *always* something to appreciate, no matter how small, even when we are struggling through a truly difficult situation. The fact it's not raining when we want our washing to dry. A car parking spot close to the supermarket (anyone else make a wish to the car-parking gods before entering the car park, or is that just me?). A cuddle with the dog. Treasure those glimmers. Notice them. Appreciate them. This is what begins to build that more positive mindset.

There is a brilliant podcast episode featuring anxiety expert Dr Jodi Richardson and Dr Helena Popovic where Dr Popovic talks about the power of having a 'Gratitude Box' in your home. Every night before dinner each family member writes down one thing they are grateful for, with their name and the date. On International Gratitude Day, 21 September, the whole family sits down and reads through all the gratitude notes. I couldn't love this more and it's something I've just started doing with my family!

I commit to finding three things I appreciate about my life every day. I will do this (when I wake/after breakfast/when I brush my teeth at night)._____.

5. HOPE

This is such a powerful emotion, and the absence of hope in our lives can be so destructive. The presence of hope is what allows us to get up in the morning, to move forward, to trust that the day will unfold as we wish. One thing I know for sure is that when we are drinking a bottle of wine (or more) most nights of the week, we certainly don't wake up with much sense of hope. In fact, most days we feel utterly hope*less*. I used to look at myself in the mirror each morning and my goodness, the names I would call myself after yet another night of drinking more than intended, waking at 3 a.m. and then tossing and turning for the next few hours. Some days I couldn't even meet my own eyes, so deep was the shame and remorse.

Calling myself useless, a failure, disgusting and pathetic was a common way for me to start my day. I have tears in my eyes as I write this. It couldn't be further from where I am today and how I speak to myself now. Waking each day full of self-loathing, remorse and disgust is not a breeding ground for positive self-talk or any sense of hope. Removing alcohol changes that.

Even in the early days of sobriety, I remember speaking to a girlfriend who asked how I was feeling now that I'd made the decision to quit for good.

I said to her, 'I know I've got work to do but I can't ignore this little fizzle in my tummy that's been there for quite some time. I've just worked out what it is. It's the feeling of hope. It's the sense that my life is about to change, get bigger. I have this really strong sense of possibility and potential for what lies ahead and, while it's foreign to me, I really, really like it!' Have you noticed that fizzle in your tummy yet?

I experience hope when I think about the future me as being _____ *and feeling* _____ .

6. AMUSEMENT

When did you last truly laugh? Those deep belly laughs that you feel in every fibre of your being? For so many of the women I coach, laughter has been missing for such a long time. We get caught up in the monotony of the day to day – the lists, the chores, the pressure and expectations that are placed on us or we place on ourselves.

It's important we find something that takes us away from that, even momentarily. For me, it's been a few different tools. The first was the podcast 'My Dad Wrote a Porno'. Now I appreciate this may not be everyone's cup of tea but, oh my, that podcast had me in fits of laughter on even the darkest and hardest days. I remember one morning when I was walking my dog having to stand on the side of the road with my legs crossed as I actually thought I was going to wet myself in public while listening to one part that had me in absolute stitches. In the midst of listening to so many serious sobriety and self-help podcasts, it was important for me to balance this out with fun and laughter. It was my little moment of 'me' time.

I make sure I spend time with the people in my life who never fail to have me in hysterics. One is my amazing friend Jo whom I travelled the world with aged 24. Every time I see or speak to her, all the memories come flooding back and she always has me in fits of laughter. Shared memories with friends is so good for the soul. I also make sure I keep up to date with the comedy shows coming to Perth for date nights and friend nights as I truly know the benefit of good, authentic belly laughs. Think about what makes you laugh, and who, and make it a priority to do more of that, or spend time regularly with that person.

I always laugh when I'm with _____ *or when I spend time doing* _____. *It's a priority for me to add this into my life and I'm going to start doing it* _____.

7. AWE

When did you last experience the emotion of awe? For me, it's always in nature. Whether I'm hiking, fishing, walking on the beach or sitting by a lake, I always take a moment to simply 'be' and take in the beauty of the natural landscape. Being in nature and taking in the shapes created in snowflakes, clouds, streams, coastlines, lakes and raindrops (known as fractals) soothes our brains and reduces stress by up to 60 per cent, according to Richard Taylor, Professor of Physics at the University of Oregon. Spend time in nature and notice the difference in your mind, stress levels and mood. It's important to note here that we have to actually look around us and not stare at the ground as we are prone to doing when walking or running. Pause, look around, and take in all the different shapes and views that Mother Nature offers.

I experience awe when I _____. *I am going to ensure I experience awe in the coming weeks by* _____

8. INSPIRATION

Who or what inspires you? Do you know? We've already talked about the impact of the five people we spend most of our time with but it's important to remember again the outcomes of being around those who inspire us. When we feel inspired, we have increased motivation to do more, be more, progress more. This is what leads to change. If we spend all our time surrounded by people who moan, blame, judge others and constantly play the victim, we are never going to feel inspired.

Pause for a moment and consider if the people in your life inspire and energise you or drain and deplete you? I came across a brilliant quote recently by Lisa Villa Prosen, author, coach and speaker on addiction recovery and personal development, which said, 'The most inspiring people I know are always evaluating and improving themselves. And the unhappiest people I know are always judging and evaluating others.' It struck a chord and resonated with me deeply. Think about who and what inspires you and carve out more time with them (these may be people you know, or who you have discovered through podcasts or TED talks). For the most inspirational people I follow, see the resources section at the back of this book.

The things and people who inspire me are _____.
I am going to dedicate more time to experiencing their inspiration by

_____.

9. JOY

What brings you joy? One definition of joy is a feeling of great pleasure and happiness. Back in my drinking days I would have answered the question about what brings me joy with 'drinking champagne with my friends'. I honestly believed that. And I'm not saying it wasn't true at the time, but it's probably the only thing I believed brought me joy. However, in sobriety, so many new aspects of life have opened up feelings of joy. Now my answer is a Sunday morning lie-in with a cup of coffee in bed and snuggles with the kids, jumping the waves with my kids at the beach, a 5-kilometre run with my dog when he speeds up for the last kilometre and pulls me up the hill, me laughing all the way, because he knows he'll get a treat at the end, a Sunday roast with my husband and kids sharing our wins for the week, a hike in the bush with girlfriends, a bubble bath with a great book and my favourite candle or an hour on the phone with one of my oldest friends in England, covering everything from our latest beauty buys to parenting dilemmas and our hacks for menopause symptoms. Joy is found in those simple moments of knowing you don't want to be anywhere else than where you are in that moment. It's those glimmers we discussed earlier. Notice what those things are for you – you may be surprised at what's been under your nose all along.

I commit to looking for and noticing five glimmers each day.

10. LOVE

Such a big and bold emotion and, when we experience it, we feel we need or want for nothing else. And I'm not only talking about romantic love here. I'm talking about love for our friends, our family, our pets and love for ourselves. Increasing self-compassion is a slow and gentle process but one that does begin to occur when we focus on ourselves, our wellbeing and our mindset. When we prioritise and look after ourselves, we are saying: 'I get to matter, I am important.' I attended a funeral recently and as I watched many people stand to share their incredibly moving eulogies of the deceased, it occurred to me how rarely we tell the people we love the most how much they mean to us. Yet when we do, it deepens and strengthens those connections tremendously. I challenge you to share with those you love how much you love them and why. When we do this, the impact is immense and the feedback incredible (and often reciprocated). Don't wait until their funeral to tell them what they mean to you.

When it comes to showing ourselves love, we can start in the most gentlest of ways. For me, that looked like starting the day by asking myself this simple question: 'How am I showing myself love today?' Try it for yourself.

EXERCISE: IDENTIFY THE POSITIVE

Consider the ten positive emotions listed on the previous pages and identify which are already abundant and present in your life and which are lacking.

Now complete the following sentence. I am going to prioritise activities and experiences that promote the feeling of _____. I will do this by adding in _____.This is important to me because _____.

Fun and happiness are free!

Something that always glaringly stands out to me when I consider the list of positive emotions is that we can experience nearly all of them without spending anything.

A walk on the beach, a podcast, a hike, reading a great book from the library, connecting with loved ones – they are all free! They are readily available and don't cost us a thing but they are never promoted or 'sold' to us because no one can make money from them. And that's where we have to be careful with the activities and other instant gratification pleasures I mentioned earlier that are being sold, advertised and marketed to us left, right and centre as the way to add more happiness to our lives. If we don't keep reminding ourselves of the ways we add true, deep joy and positivity to our lives and set clear intentions of how we are going to implement them, we become vulnerable to believing what the big food, alcohol, tech and consumer companies tell us will bring us happiness.

The advertising strategy of major companies to ensure we buy their products is to induce FUD – 'fear, uncertainty and doubt'. Everywhere we look messages are being thrown at us that if we don't purchase a particular product we will have a 'less than' life. Of course, there isn't any advertising anywhere that focuses on time cuddling your kids or walking in nature. There's no money to be made out of that! When we become aware of this, we can start to notice the difference between things we are sold that give us short-term pleasure and the things that bring us natural joy.

EXERCISE: MAKE A LIST

If you know that your fun plan is missing a few vital pieces, try these journal prompts to open your mind and way of thinking when it comes to adding in fun.

☐ Who are the people in your life with whom you always have a great time, no matter what you're doing? Fun can be a person as much as an activity. (I've worked on a pumpkin farm polishing pumpkins for twelve hours a day and look back at it being one of the most fun times of my life, based on the brilliant people in that pumpkin shed with me!).

☐ Make a list of the people who make you feel great when you spend time with them, and arrange to see them again. Know who energises you and who drains you – and spend time with those energisers!

☐ Make a bucket list of 30 things you'd love to do in the next ten years. Go crazy with this! Don't hold back – you might want to walk the Inca trail, travel in a hot air balloon, sing on stage in front of a live audience, write a book, ride a horse at sunset on the beach, watch a Broadway musical, learn a musical instrument. The list is endless – only your imagination holds you back! Pin it on your fridge to keep reminding yourself of your dreams. And then make them happen!

☐ What have you said 'no' to in the last ten years that you wished you had said 'yes' to but fear, time or money held you back? That's a great clue as to what you might like to do.

☐ Who or what are you jealous of? Jealousy is a great clue to discovering what we might want in our lives. Don't shy away from this emotion – embrace it and use it as a tool of self-discovery.

Developing healthy, happy habits

Before we end this chapter, I want to share with you my top ten healthy, happy habits. These are the small steps I take each day to improve my mental and emotional wellbeing which have helped me reach the point where I no longer want, or need, to drink. Remember, your mental and emotional wellbeing is influenced by all the decisions you make each day, such as the foods you eat, how you spend your time, who you spend it with, whether you exercise, whether you prioritise sleep. All these things impact how positive your mindset will be.

As we have discussed, when we take alcohol out of our lives, we have to add new habits in. Listed opposite are mine. Try them and see for yourself if they lift your mood and, like me, lead you to feeling a deeper sense of contentment, peace and joy at the end of the day.

Movement and exercise (for those endorphin hits!).	Connection with a friend or family member – in person or on the phone.
Getting nature hits by spending some time outside being present in the natural world.	Limiting time on social media and being intentional with who I follow, only following people who truly inspire me.
Eating foods that promote serotonin production (as outlined in Chapter 4).	Listening to music. Morning breakfast dance parties with the kids are a great way to start the day!
Offering acts of kindness and service, such as helping an elderly lady with her shopping or letting someone into the queue ahead of me. Helping others improves our own sense of wellbeing. It's a win-win.	Having a creative outlet where I enter a flow state, such as cooking, writing, reading, running, decluttering, jigsawing (no, it's not a word but it is now!).
Practising self-care, saying 'I matter' and dedicating a small amount of time to me each day – a bath, a walk, a meditation, yoga, a sauna.	Treasuring the glimmers and joyful experiences, aiming for five a day – noticing them and saying a silent word of gratitude.

EXERCISE: PICKING HEALTHY HABITS

What would you pick out of the habits above, or what haven't I included that you would add in?

Consider what you do in your current day that you don't really enjoy, and brainstorm ways you could delegate, say no or create a boundary in order to free up time to add in some of the more joyful activities we have discussed.

Here are some examples:

ACTIVITY I DON'T ENJOY OR WASTE TIME ON	HOW I COULD CHANGE THIS	WHAT I COULD DO WITH THIS TIME
Social media scrolling	Set boundaries around social media time	Meditate or read
Food shopping and meal prepping	Online food orders, get family involved in meal prepping and delegate three nights a week	Try a night class learning something new such as bridge.
Driving the kids to activities every afternoon	Carpool with other parents or use the time I am there to do something else	Walk while kids are at sport and listen to an audio book or podcast
Housework every Saturday	Create a roster in the family to delegate and put it on the fridge	Saturday morning yoga and coffee with a friend
Ironing most nights	Delegate, investigate ironing services or try hanging in a way ironing is minimised	Have a bath and read or listen to music

Onwards!

My hope is that you have begun to redefine what fun and happiness mean for you and that I've given you some ideas of ways to incorporate these into your life, without alcohol. It's essential we do this to ensure we don't feel like we are missing out and instead continue to feed those positive emotions. Boredom is real in middle-aged women and it's our job to ensure we are taking the steps to mitigate this and add in fun elements where we can.

This is *your* opportunity to live the fullest and most fun-filled life possible!

SOBER ACTION STEPS

☐ Redefine your own fun plan and consider activities you do or would like to do that are simply for your pleasure.

☐ Consider where the positive emotions feature in your life and where they are lacking so you can take steps to ensure you experience them more.

☐ Be aware of the instant gratification activities that rob us of time, money and energy, and instead look for and notice the glimmers.

☐ Write your own bucket list – I bet you'll be surprised by what comes up for you. Get the family involved too!

☐ Delegate and plan ahead so you make sure each week you include the activities you love.

SOBER SISTERS

SARAH

Ever since I was a teenager I dabbled in alcohol and drugs. In my late 20s and early 30s, I stopped drinking as much while I had my two children. But after separating from their father, alcohol became a routine. I drank when I was sad. Stressed. Had a hard day. Celebrating. Alcohol became my new friend. A way to numb myself.

After more than a decade of drowning my sorrows, I'd put on 12 kilograms, my hair was falling out to the point where I was googling wigs, my face was bloated, eyes dead, I had high blood pressure and was inexplicably and perpetually anxious. But still every evening I'd look forward to that first drink. My treat, my reward for making it through another hard day as a working solo parent.

I didn't have a 'rock bottom' moment that made me reconsider my relationship with alcohol in my 40s. I was just sick and tired of feeling sick and tired. Initially, I decided to go 100 days without alcohol. But once the 100 days finished, I started drinking on the weekends again. I quickly returned to autopilot, drinking almost every night at the same level I had been before. When my mum was diagnosed with a rare aggressive cancer, I hit the bottle even harder. She survived only mere months. I feel deep regret that the night she passed away I'd had so many drinks I had to get a lift to the hospice to be by her side. I wasn't fully present for her when she was at her most vulnerable. After her tragic death at such a young age, I knew I wanted more from my one life. I knew I was capable of more. And I knew I had to do something different if I wanted to permanently ditch booze.

I realised the biggest secret to sobriety is that simply ditching alcohol isn't enough. You need to add things in if you want a life that brings you joy.

I now use my newfound energy and oodles of free time to get my dopamine hits from dance classes. I loved ballet and contemporary dance well into my late teens. And guess what, I still love it in my 40s! I do Pilates every Saturday morning with a friend and then we have a coffee. I lift weights three times a week. I walk the dog morning and evening and, rather than keeping my sad and sorry head down, I love chatting to the people I come across. When I cook dinner, I throw on some tunes and bop around. My house is cleaner. I love cooking nourishing food.

I take time to do things that are true self-care, from simple gestures like a bubble bath to taking time away from the kids to go to a retreat or a long hike in the middle of nowhere overseas. I am now positively modelling to my children that I matter, my time matters and that I have dreams and desires that go beyond the daily slog of parenthood.

I've made so many more real genuine connections than I ever did when I was drinking heavily. I choose to spend time with friends who are authentic, who share similar values, whose presence fuels me. My confidence has skyrocketed. I socialise now more than ever and have even been sober raving and rocked it out in the mosh pit.

I have created a life I don't want to numb myself from.

CHAPTER 9
VALUE YOUR LIFE!
Creating a life that prioritises what you love

A while back, I was working with a client who had been signed off work with depression. Her anxiety, and therefore her drinking, had increased and she had lost interest and motivation in her job, her family and, honestly, her whole life. She felt confused and scared. While she wasn't clinically depressed, she felt deeply out of sorts and not herself, and she couldn't work out why.

Over time and through some initial sessions, I gained insight into her life leading up to this time. We talked about her career and her previous drinking, which was very standard with no signs of alcohol use disorder prior to recent months, and we finally came to the realisation that she was living so out of alignment with her core values that it was hugely impacting her mental wellbeing and driving her to drink more as a result. This was showing up through cultural changes at work that directly contradicted her work ethic and morals, forcing her to act with clients in a way that she wasn't comfortable with and she felt lacked integrity. It was also leading to longer working hours and seeing less of her family, rarely being home in time to put her kids to bed and then drinking heavily most evenings to switch off.

Yet the fact was, my client didn't realise that this lack of alignment with her values was the issue, as she didn't even know what her core values were, let alone know she was out of alignment with them. All she knew was she felt withdrawn, low and emotional, and was drinking much more as a way to escape those emotions.

This is such a common scenario for many women and is why 'values' work is so instrumental to our journey of self-discovery and creating a more fulfilling and joyful life. Common symptoms of not living aligned to our values include feelings of anxiety, depression, withdrawal, incessant rage and anger, regret and resentment. I would go so far as to say that understanding and reconnecting with core values is one of the most influential and important exercises we can do. When we know our values and we create a life aligned to them, everything feels easier and calmer.

Do you know your core values, and how well aligned to your life they are?

What do you value?

Our values are what matter to us, what we place importance on in all aspects of our lives, in how we show up, in our work, in our families and in our communities.

We are all different and we all value different things. While there's no right or wrong when it comes to values, it is important that we know and understand our personal values, as every decision we make in our lives can be positively or negatively impacted depending on whether it is aligned with them. One of the simplest and most effective ways of improving our wellbeing is to live congruently with our values. But we can't do that if we don't what they are!

If we clearly know our values, we have a sense of purpose in life and can move towards our goals because we know what matters most to us. Knowing my values influences every decision I make and also provides clues for when I might not be on my right path. When I am living in alignment with my values I am showing up as my most authentic self. I feel calm, content, light and joyful – like everything is 'right'.

Equally, when I am out of alignment with my values, I always know. How? For me this shows up physically – a sense of unease, a knot forming in my tummy, anger rising in my chest, withdrawing from a conversation or meeting, or ruminating over something I said or did for some time after the event. I also have increased anxiety and trouble sleeping.

Any time we are out of alignment with our values, we are out of alignment with our core, authentic selves and this is when issues can arise.

Yet so many of us live for so long (perhaps forever!) without ever knowing our values, and that is because alcohol nearly always takes us away from living a life aligned to them.

Do your words and actions match up?

When I was drinking, nearly all my core values were so heavily compromised that I was in complete misalignment. I valued family and yet I ignored my children so I could drink. I valued my health and yet I consumed at least four times the recommended amount of alcohol a week. I valued authenticity and yet I was loose-lipped and indiscreet after a bottle of wine. I valued adventure and yet my life was so small, doing the same things week in and week out, afraid to try anything new. I valued service to others and yet I couldn't even volunteer to help at the school canteen as I was often too hungover on a Friday morning. I valued learning but I was too 'exhausted' (i.e. hungover) to spend any time learning anything. And I valued connection, yet I wasn't connecting on a deep, authentic level in the way I do now in sobriety.

As I'm sure you can imagine, the impact this had on my mental health was huge. I wasn't showing up as the mum, friend, wife or community member I wanted to be. And I wasn't showing up as the version of *me* I wanted to be. I didn't even know who I was. In so many ways, removing alcohol was the single first step to begin living a life aligned to my values. And I know I have said this many times but please let me say it again: this is our one and only life so we need to make the absolute most of it.

I have supported women aged from 25 to 75 to remove alcohol, make significant changes in their life and reap the benefits. And so often this starts with making the decision to take a break from alcohol, discover their values and then take steps to live more aligned with them. It makes us feel whole again, often at a time when we feel so disconnected and fragmented.

As author and founder of the Be Sober online community Simon Chapple says in his book, *How to Heal Your Inner Child*:

> Your values are unique to you, and if you live your life in line with them, they will act as a compass, keeping you on track for a happy life and ensuring that you spend your time engaging in the things that bring you joy and meet your needs.

I invite you to consider for a moment how you feel in your day-to-day life. Do you feel calm and content? Do you feel that you are on track to moving towards your goals? Do you end each day feeling proud and fulfilled with a deep sense of self connection? If not, you are most likely out of alignment with your values and the following exercise will be a powerful tool for you.

EXERCISE: VALUE YOURSELF

1. Take a moment of silence to connect into yourself. Perhaps do a short meditation or ten rounds of deep breathing. Something that grounds you and quietens the 'noise' because it's important the following comes from your soul, not your thinking/working brain.

2. Remove any 'shoulds'. This is not about selecting values you think you 'should' have. There is absolutely no right or wrong. Your values are unique to you and you alone.

3. Circle all the words/values in the table opposite that resonate with you as being important in how you show up in life and what you value in other people.

4. Next, create five columns and group the values you've selected into each column according to which feel the most similar to you.

5. Look at each column and pick the one word that stands out as being the 'leader' for that column. At the end you will have five core values.

6. Reflect on the values by asking yourself:

☐ Am I in alignment with this value right now?

☐ What's one step I could take to be more aligned to this value?

☐ When I am not aligned to this value, I feel _____.

Ability	Diligence	Imagination	Routine
Abundance	Discipline	Independence	Security
Acceptance	Discretion	Ingenuity	Self-actualisation
Accountability	Diversity	Inner harmony	Self-control
Accuracy	Dynamism	Innovation	Selflessness
Achievement	Economy	Inquisitiveness	Self-regulation
Adventurousness	Effectiveness	Insightfulness	Self-reliance
Altruism	Efficiency	Intelligence	Sensitivity
Ambition	Elegance	Intellectual status	Serenity
Approachability	Empathy	Intuition	Service
Assertiveness	Enjoyment	Joy	Shrewdness
Autonomy	Enthusiasm	Justice	Simplicity
Balance	Equality	Knowledge	Soundness
Being the best	Excellence	Leadership	Speed
Belonging	Excitement	Learning	Spontaneity
Boldness	Expertise	Legacy	Stability
Calmness	Exploration	Love	Strategic
Carefulness	Expressiveness	Loyalty	Strength
Challenge	Fairness	Making a difference	Structure
Cheerfulness	Faith	Mastery	Success
Clear-minded	Family-oriented	Merit	Support
Commitment	Fidelity	Obedience	Teamwork
Community	Fitness	Openness	Temperance
Compassion	Flexibility	Optimism	Thankfulness
Competence	Fluency	Order	Thoroughness
Competitiveness	Focus	Originality	Thoughtfulness
Consistency	Freedom	Patriotism	Timeliness
Contentment	Friendship	Perfection	Tolerance
Continuous improvement	Fun	Piety	Traditionalism
Contribution	Generosity	Positivity	Trustworthiness
Control	Goodness	Practicality	Truth
Cooperation	Grace	Preparedness	Understanding
Correctness	Growth	Prestige	Uniqueness
Courage	Happiness	Professionalism	Unity
Courtesy	Hard work	Prudence	Usefulness
Creativity	Harmony	Quality-oriented	Valiance
Curiosity	Health	Reliability	Variety
Decisiveness	Helping society	Resilience	Vision
Democratic	Holiness	Resourcefulness	Vitality
Dependability	Honesty	Restraint	Zeal
Determination	Honour	Results-oriented	Zest
Devoutness	Humility	Rigour	

SOBRIETY IS ...

'The "me" I always wanted to be but
never thought I'd get there. '

DANIELLE

'Giving me the freedom me to
express all the parts of myself I've
kept hidden and numb with alcohol.
I am finally free!'

KATE

'Feeling so much more confident,
capable, smarter,
brave, and calm.'

JESSICA

Living your values

Remember, these are your values and no one else's. Once you know them you can make every decision in your life based on whether it takes you closer to your values or away from them.

Stick your values somewhere you see them every day – the fridge, bedroom mirror, above your desk – so they become an integral part of *you*.

Something that has served me well over the last few years is having my values written somewhere I see them every day. This way I am constantly reminded of them and when I set myself small goals and intentions for the week ahead, the list will ensure I am in alignment with my values.

For example:

- **Family**: I ensure we have five meals a week together at the dinner table with no TV or screens.

- **Connection**: I arrange quality time with friends.

- **Health**: I set goals around my fitness and mental wellbeing (meditation, journaling, etc.).

- **Service**: I conduct at least one act of service a week, whether it be helping a neighbour with some shopping or delivering a free talk on my Instagram account on ways to address grey area drinking.

Setting these intentions and checking in with them is super helpful and ensures I feel really good through the week. How could you set yours?

Developing an 'operating system'

Next, it is useful to begin to develop our own unique operating system, which can support us to create a life that is in alignment with our core values. Consider your operating system to be the foundations that support your mental, physical and emotional wellbeing and, for the most part, become your non-negotiables for how you live your life. When we know what makes us feel good, we need to make sure we keep doing those things. Once again, this comes back to us being *present* in our lives, aware of what does and doesn't make us feel our best, what needs to stay and what we need to remove.

While our mental wellbeing, mood and mindset are dependent on many factors at play in any given moment (such as hormones, other people and external circumstances, for example), I know for sure that when I live my life with my operating system working optimally, everything in my life is better and my mental health is at its absolute best. My thoughts are clearer and more positive, I am more confident, I feel more connected. I feel in alignment with my values and I feel calm. Consider your operating system your blueprint to creating your strongest emotional and mental wellbeing.

The actions in my operation system are the things I *can* control in a world where so many things feel completely *out* of control, something we have already talked about so much in this book. They are my way of prioritising myself and my needs.

Any time I find myself feeling more anxious, my thoughts becoming more negative or self-sabotaging behaviours creeping in, I simply take a look at my operating system and can quickly see when and where a few things might have dropped off.

Now I don't always live my life in alignment with this system 100 per cent of the time but I do aim for 80 per cent most days. It's helped me massively and I hope in sharing my system with you, it helps you to create your own.

There can be as many facets as you like but I recommend no more than twelve, or else it can look and feel overwhelming. What goes on the operating system are the things you know enhance and improve your mental and emotional wellbeing (and if you're not sure of that yet, start by using mine and then as you go on, decide whether or not to keep them).

MY OPERATING SYSTEM

The following priorities make up my personal operating system, which also includes a table that I use to tick each action off (see page 222). Just to be clear, I don't tick off everything every single day but aim to complete about 80 per cent.

Eight hours of sleep, bed by 10 p.m. latest

We have already learnt how important sleep is for our physical and mental wellbeing. I know being tired is a primary factor for me indulging in any self-sabotaging behaviour such as mindless scrolling, eating junk, not exercising and negative thought patterns. Prioritising my sleep plays a huge role in my positive mental wellbeing.

Connection to self

This can take the form of meditation, journaling, breath work, affirmations and visualising the day ahead (rarely all of these but always at least one). These acts of quieting my mind and going inward (instead of always being on alert, looking outward) means I check in with myself to monitor how I'm doing and what I need in any given moment. My 6 a.m. morning routine is essential to my wellbeing. If you're interested in creating your own morning routine, I highly recommend the book *The Miracle Morning* by Hal Elrod.

Alcohol-free

There are some days where the shit hits the fan and nothing goes to plan. That's life, right? But one thing I know for sure is that every single night when my head hits the pillow, I can be proud and grateful that I chose not to drink. I will never not be proud of my sobriety, even when I'm 30 years sober, and nor should you!

Movement

Walking, yoga, swimming, biking, ideally outside in nature. As we've already discussed, movement of any kind is such a fundamental factor in our mental wellbeing, causing us to get a surge of the supportive neurotransmitters dopamine and serotonin, a dose of vitamin D if we are outside, and raising our heart rate. Even just getting out for a walk does more than I bet you even realise! What could be the first starting point for you? A ten-minute walk when you get home from work? A yoga class two nights a week?

Six to eight servings of a combination of veg, fruit, legumes a day

The more I learn about the link between nutrition and mental wellbeing, anxiety and menopause symptoms, the more I focus on my diet and what

I choose to put in my mouth. I have begun prioritising adding many more vegetables and legumes (beans, peas, lentils) into my diet. Fun fact: beans are a great source of soluble fibre, which means they draw toxins out of our bile duct so we excrete them rather than have them circulating around our body, which can make us feel pretty awful – both mentally and physically.

Since adding extra beans to my diet and prioritising fresh fruit and vegetables over other food I have noticed the following awesome changes: weight loss, fewer sugar cravings (I can literally look at a piece of chocolate cake and not even *want* it!), less bloating, improved energy, improved digestion, better sleep and improved mental health and mood. A cup of beans a day (either black, kidney, mung, borlotti, lentils or chickpeas) have become a non-negotiable for me. If I go a few days without beans, I really notice the difference in my body and my mind.

In-person connection with my tribe

As we have already explored in Chapter 6, connection with people in real life is so important. In a world that is becoming more and more disconnected, isolated and navigated through devices, adding in real-life connection soothes our soul and our nervous system and fills our cup with love, authenticity and joy. Prioritise face-to-face time with the people you love. Humans were built for real-life connection, not staying connected via sending each other TikToks and Instagram reels once a week (which has definitely been known to happen in my friendship circle during times of busy craziness). Set an intention to see and touch your loved ones, not just send them messages.

Screen-free connection time with my family

As a mum to a tween and teenager there is a constant battle to set limits for screen time and ensuring time off devices. I recall my daughter saying, 'Mum, you are constantly telling me to get off the iPad and yet you are always on your phone.' Ouch! She was right. (Isn't it often said that our kids are our greatest teachers?!)

Setting boundaries around screen time and ensuring we have authentic connection each day is fundamental to my core family values. We try to eat together every night but it's not always possible with various kids' activities so I have a few extra ways to get this time together, such as doing jigsaw puzzles (with my daughter), walks and kicking rugby goals (with my son), beach walks and swims every Sunday morning (family), baking and cooking (both kids), chats in the car with no screens (I have the best chats with my son on our car journeys). Ensuring this ongoing connection is crucial as they get older. My hubby and I prioritise evening walks several times a week, weekly saunas and those rituals of connection I talked about in Chapter 6.

Self-growth

Every day I read or listen to something that inspires me. As we have already talked about, being curious and feeling inspired are key positive emotions and ones we can seek out each day, in a way that doesn't have to impact too much on our daily lives. I often listen to a podcast in the car or when walking or cleaning or I read when I'm waiting for the kids to finish sport (instead of scrolling on my phone). I have a seemingly endless list of books and podcasts to finish (and that list just seems to get longer – yours, too?!) but none of it feels like a chore because they all spark my interest and make me want to explore further. There is no right or wrong; it's just about listening to your own clues of what interests you and following them. But the key here is to listen, be curious and notice what sparks interest. Give yourself space to do this by not filling every spare moment with mindless scrolling, which I know I was guilty of for so long.

Self-care activity just for me

As we have discussed, nervous system regulation and managing stress are the foundation for so many of us to not even *want* to pick up a drink. This starts with self-care and prioritising our own needs, as we discussed in Chapter 5. Rather than just *think* about what you want to do for yourself, I encourage you to plan and organise the things you *will* do for yourself.

In fact, I would go so far as to say, start each day with deciding the one thing that you will do for *you* that day. An evening bath with your favourite book? Half an hour with a recipe book to plan a meal for the weekend, a yoga class, an online sound healing class, fifteen minutes of stretching, an early night? As we already know, it doesn't have to be big grand gestures as it's simply not practical to plan a massage, facial, reiki and a breathwork session each day! But these smaller acts of self-care are equally as important because they are a way of saying 'I matter'.

ACTIVITY	MON	TUES	WED	THURS	FRI	SAT	SUN
Eight hours sleep							
Movement/ exercise							
Time outside							
Screen-free time with family							
Self-care activity just for me							
In-person connection with friend/s							
Connection to self (journaling, meditation)							
Alcohol-free							
Six to eight servings of fruit, veg or legumes							
Learning and self-growth							
Limit screen time to two hours a day, phone off 8 p.m.							

LET'S REFLECT

Now it's your turn. What might be in your operating system? What are the things that you know make you feel your absolute best?

Complete these sentences:

I know when I _____, _____, and _____ (insert three things you know improve or enhance your life in some way) I feel _____.
It's important to me to prioritise time to do these because _____. My first step is to _____.

Redefining success

What were you taught success was when you were growing up? I expect that like many of us born in the post-war era, success was measured by your possessions and the state of your finances: owning a home, what car you drive, where you go on holiday and what your job title is. But what if instead of measuring success by these material outcomes, we measured it by a feeling? How would you answer the question of what success is then?

If I ask you, 'How do you want to *feel* at the end of the week' or 'How do you want to *feel* in ten years' time?' I am sure not many of you would answer: 'Stressed, exhausted, frazzled, overwhelmed, hungover or disillusioned.' And yet that is what I see so many people feel when they are chasing the goals of material possessions. Prior to commencing my role as a grey area drinking and health and wellness coach, I worked for 23 years as an executive recruiter, primarily in the legal and banking sectors. I supported some of the wealthiest individuals I've ever met to make their next career move and I can honestly tell you, most of them weren't happy and didn't experience much joy in their lives. They were burnt out, overwhelmed and always worried that their performance would drop and the rug would be pulled from beneath them at any moment. When all we do is aim for financial or status goals we rarely achieve authentic joy and happiness.

When I ask my clients 'How do you want to feel at the end of the week, this time next year?' the majority of responses are, 'Content, peaceful, free, calm, relaxed, joyful and with space to think.' And I don't think any of us achieve this at the end of a 60-hour work week. But what I found was that when I was living according to my operating system, ensuring my life included activities that calmed and soothed me, as well as activities and people who lit me up and inspired me, feelings of peace, contentment, fulfilment and joy were all within reach.

Let's start measuring success by feelings and not external goals.

The feeling of success comes as a result of creating a life with more purpose.

What is my purpose in life and how do I find it?

I remember pondering this question so much back in 2019 when I'd first removed alcohol. I had this newfound energy, more time, more clarity and a feeling that I wanted to fulfil myself more but I had no idea where to start. Little did I know that just a few short years later I'd have the privilege of supporting thousands of women to change their lives, which would lead me here, to writing this book.

I can truly say I have found my purpose and I live it every day, and I want to touch on ways that you can experience this, too. This doesn't mean you have to change anything as huge as your job, home and/or country but I will guide you through some questions that helped me when I was pondering this very subject.

The Oxford Dictionary offers two useful definitions for the concept of 'purpose'. The first is 'the reason for which something is done or created or for which something exists', and the second is 'a person's sense of resolve or determination'. If we put this into the context of our entire life, this makes sense to me – purpose is the reason we exist and our sense of determination.

When we wake each morning with a plan to do the things we love and place value and importance on, we have a sense of purpose, a reason to jump out of bed and go about our day with a spring in our step. If we don't have any sense of purpose, it makes sense that we might struggle, feel demotivated, flat and low in mood, and become easily sidetracked with activities and pastimes that entice us but don't necessarily fulfil us (such as alcohol, social media or online shopping).

This isn't to say we can, or should, all have hugely purposeful lives and everything we do should offer us great joy and purpose (although how amazing would that be!). There are always going to be some things we do in life that we find more joy and importance in than others. That's life. But it's essential that we find a balance, because life without our fun activities, joys and valued pastimes can feel meaningless and more likely to keep us reaching for the bottle to escape.

While it would be lovely to create a life that was 100 per cent purposeful and meaningful, it just isn't practical for most. We often can't leave our jobs to go hiking with the silver-back gorillas in the Ugandan jungle for months on end or live on the *Sea Shepherd* defending marine wildlife. But we can ensure that we are intentional with how we spend our time *outside* of the things we don't get as much meaning from. Enter the rise of the slash career!

We don't have to be defined just by the job we do. We don't have to only refer to ourselves as nurses, teachers, retailers or marketing managers. We can be defined as much for the unpaid, but often more meaningful, activities that we do outside of work! Here is where the slash career comes in. I have clients who are nurses/photographers, teachers/singers, retailers/jewellery makers, admin managers/ musicians and project managers/writers.

What would be your slash career? What/who are you outside of your job? And while many of you may say, 'mothers, cleaners, Uber drivers, cooks, bed makers and dog walkers', I would love you to dive a little deeper outside of the roles you have as CEOs of little people and running the home. I know how time-consuming these roles are but it's so important we have something more outside of being a mother, wife, worker and home runner. If we don't, we run the risk of feeling extremely lost and disheartened when children leave home, or when unexpected redundancies or retirement happen.

Still feeling stuck with what your slash career might be? The following exercise may help.

LET'S REFLECT

Use these questions to think about what you could be doing more of or adding into your life to create more purpose.

1. What's that thing you can do that makes you lose track of time and forget to go to the loo, check your phone or eat your lunch?

2. What did you love doing as a child? What would you be found doing for hours on end, when there wasn't Candy Crush or Facebook to entertain us?

3. When you are feeling most alive, most at one with yourself, what are you doing?

4. What can't you keep quiet about? What would cause you to speak up, step in or take over if you saw this thing happening?

5. If you knew you had one year left on this earth, what would you simply *have* to do and experience?

6. What did you want to be when you grew up?

7. What's one thing you would love to start doing or continue doing that you'd love to still be doing on your last day on earth?

8. When you wake in the morning and consider your day ahead, which activities or experiences do you place the most importance on or feel the most joy from?

The path to success

Now that we have established what our values are and begun to live in alignment with them, we have an operating system that ensures our mental and emotional wellbeing is optimal, and we regularly participate in activities and experiences that are important to us, we are on the path to creating a life filled with contentment and ease.

We soften and relax, knowing that we are exactly where we are meant to be, doing exactly what we are meant to be doing. It's a wonderful feeling! And one that is entirely within reach for all of us, when we make the decision to reflect, explore, tweak and add *in* to our own unique and incredible lives. And that's exactly what I knew I wanted – not to simply *exist* but to *live* and have a wonderful, crazy, wild and challenging life that brings joy each day.

SOBER ACTION STEPS

☐ Discover your values and assess where you might be out of alignment with them. Establish the first step to living more in alignment.

☐ Create your own unique operating system that includes all your personal non-negotiables, so you know you are on track to protecting and enhancing your physical, mental and emotional wellbeing.

☐ Consider your own slash career. Journal on the questions I've posed and discover what may have been suppressed inside you for so long that is just waiting to jump out!

☐ Give yourself full permission to follow these steps, knowing it's what is required to ensure you're creating, and living, your best life, without the need or desire for any alcohol whatsoever.

ELLIE

I had always used alcohol to become the 'party girl' growing up. However, after a messy divorce, my relationship with alcohol shifted from the merely social to the medicinal, to help with stress, sleep, just to switch off.

By the time my children had grown up I was habitually drinking a bottle of wine a night, maybe more, by myself. When I remarried, my new husband asked me many times to cut down but I took that as a criticism and it hardened my resolve to continue to drink: it was my life, after all.

My drinking didn't just impact me; it impacted everyone around me. And I didn't see the damage I was doing to my family. I was irrational, argumentative and extremely selfish. I was the worst possible role model for my adult children.

There was no 'rock bottom' moment that led me to stop. I just woke up one day and decided enough was enough. To be honest, I was surprised at how easy it was to stop. But I think what made it easier was the sudden clarity I had about what it was taking from me.

To start with I avoided social occasions. I wanted to be secure in my sobriety before I tested myself. When I did go out, I rang ahead to see what alcohol-free options were available. I visualised how I would respond to people's questions (I decided on the blunt 'I had a hugely dysfunctional relationship with alcohol, it needed to stop before it killed me'), and I avoided situations I felt would be triggering. I gradually added fun and meaningful things back into my life. I made myself accountable to as many people as I could.

But the biggest strategy for success was to surround myself with an understanding support network of other women following the same path.

Alcohol at the time was my go-to in times of stress. I can see now it was doing me no favours and, as a method of stress-relief, was scientifically flawed! A long walk with the dogs in the forest is so much more calming, as is a soak in a hot bath, or a walk on the beach at dusk. I have done yoga for the first time in my life. Self-talk has been my lifesaver, taking myself to a place of calm and quiet and giving myself space to think through stressful situations.

I have always been organised, with a life plan, but alcohol meant it was always sabotaged by procrastination. I had dreams but they were blurry, seemingly unobtainable. Since removing alcohol, I have embarked on a course to train as a nutrition and wellbeing coach. It has filled the gap left by the fog of alcohol very effectively both by giving me something physical to do in the evenings, and also fuelling my awakened brain with knowledge.

On an emotional level, stopping drinking has been a bit of a roller-coaster. All the feelings I didn't know I had blocked out, all my perceived inadequacies, the hurts, the regrets, as well as the massive guilt from all the times I messed up under the influence, came flooding back in. But moving forward I have learnt to sit in serenity with myself and, with a clear and now objective outlook on life, there is more balance and more equilibrium.

Happiness and the happiness of my family is my priority and is not negotiable. Authenticity and being true to my values is paramount. My wellbeing is important: self-esteem, mindfulness, health and, of course, sobriety are the catalysts for change and the scaffolding on which my future rests. This is my gift to myself and to my children.

I am not prepared to accept a life half-lived. I want to be the best possible version of myself.

YOUR 'HAPPILY EVER AFTER'

So here we are, at the end of the book, but more importantly, at the beginning of your new life.

As I'm sure you have come to realise from all that you have read, the journey of sobriety isn't really about alcohol at all. That's perhaps 10 per cent of the process. The other 90 per cent is what we do differently with our health, time, relationships and mindset. It's about creating a new identity. Becoming the type of woman who looks after herself, listens to herself, prioritises herself and finally, who loves herself in full technicolour glory.

Before we close, let's recap what have become my five foundational pillars of sobriety. I hope these help you no matter where you are on your journey.

Remember, the journey of self-discovery is not quick, nor is it easy. However, continuing to drink isn't easy either.

> Sobriety gets easier with time, and life, most definitely, gets richer.

1. FACE YOUR REASONS FOR DRINKING

Use the tools in this book to identify why you drink. This is a crucial first step in addressing the issue. Common reasons include stress, boredom and loneliness. What problems, feelings or unconscious thoughts are you masking with alcohol? Becoming aware of what lies behind your drinking can unlock the path to change.

2. SAY *YES* TO DOING THINGS DIFFERENTLY

It doesn't work if you remove alcohol but keep everything else in your life the same. You have to change other aspects, too. You have to add *in* when you take alcohol *out*. This might mean saying *yes* to adding in new hobbies, courses, activities and experiences that will enrich and add to your life. Say *yes* to looking after your body through your sleep, nutrition, exercise and stress management routine. It might also mean some tough conversations but if we avoid them we remain unhappy. Say *yes* to yourself, which sometimes might mean saying *no* to others.

3. CONNECTION IS KEY

Being able to connect with people as our true, authentic self is essential. I find the sober community a wonderful place for creating these connections, so you may like to start there. I have a warm and beautiful community of women who will welcome you with open arms, 'The Women's Wellbeing Collective' on Facebook. As one of my clients said to me in her recent feedback survey: 'For the first time in 54 years, I have felt seen.' Think quality over quantity when it comes to connecting. Find the right people and love them hard.

4. TELL YOUR STORY AND BE OF SERVICE

When I began sharing my story about my journey to sobriety, I found it gave other women hope. In sharing my story, I was helping them. Consider the smallest of ways you can be of service. Support women new to sobriety, share your own story, speak up, don't be afraid to challenge the status quo and go against the norm. If you can do it, others can do it, too.

5. TAKE RESPONSIBILITY FOR YOUR LIFE

One of the most important messages I hope you will take from this book is that *your life is 100 per cent your responsibility*. It's no one else's job to make you happy, stop you being so bored, or make new friends appear by magic in front of you. Only you can do that. It's up to you to create the life you want. And that starts with *knowing* what you want and then taking steps to get there. 'I want more connection' means we take steps to join groups or community gatherings where we can meet more people. 'I want more energy' means we look at nutrition, exercise and lifestyle factors. 'I want time to explore activities just for me' means we set boundaries and make a commitment to researching and experiencing new activities. It's only ever up to us to make the effort to create the life we want.

Above all else, remember that the process of creating a happy, fulfilling and joyful alcohol-free life does take time. It's also not just about reaching the destination – it's about what we experience along the way. That is where the growth and self-discovery happen.

Most importantly, focus on what you're gaining, not what you're missing, and you'll start to experience your life in full, technicolour glory!

What do I consider the greatest benefits of sobriety? It's the sense of pride I have for waking up every day alcohol-free in a world where alcohol is pushed, sold and promoted everywhere I turn. It's the energy and mental clarity I now have which has allowed me to explore, experiment and create a life I love. It's the connection to my loved ones, the modelling I'm doing for my kids, the depth of connection I now have with my husband and most importantly, the connection I have with myself. For the first time in my life, I can look myself in the mirror every morning and give myself a little wink while whispering the words, 'I love you and I'm proud of you.' What's not to love about that? Never underestimate the impact that removing alcohol can have on every aspect of your life, not just your liver health. Removing alcohol is the greatest act of self-care you can show yourself and is the single most effective way to give you the biggest bang for your buck when it comes to impact on your life!

Finally, what do you *really* want? Picture yourself a year from now, five years from now, ten years from now. If nothing at all has changed, how does that make you feel? And now consider the following questions: 'How do you really want to feel? How do you want to be showing up in your life? Who do you want to be?' It's all there for the taking – we just have to believe we are worth it. And to acknowledge that alcohol isn't the route to getting it – in fact, it will only take us in the opposite direction. I believe in you. The question is, do *you* believe in you? I truly hope so.

I invite you to commit to being the new you. Complete this sentence for the future you.

I am the type of person who _____

_____.

Please do email me your response to that sentence. I absolutely *love* hearing from you.

Remember,
I see you,
I honour you,
I am you.

Huge love,

Sarah Rusbatch

xxxxx

SPECIAL THANKS

When I was a little girl, I would lock myself away for hours on end writing story after story. And if I wasn't writing, I was reading. Books have been a part of my life for so long and it was always a dream to one day write my own book. To have had the opportunity to do this, and for it to be because of the decision I made in April 2019 to remove alcohol from my life, will always be one of my greatest achievements (after my children and my sobriety).

I'm sure it won't surprise you to know that turning dreams into reality takes time, effort, commitment, belief and support. And for the endless support I have been blessed to receive, I want to share my gratitude. The first thanks goes to my incredible mentor Kathy Rhodes. At the end of 2022 Kathy asked me what my dream was for 2023. I told her, 'I have a lifelong dream to write a book, but I don't see how that's going to happen.' Without even a blink of the eye Kathy said, 'Let's make sure it does happen. What's our first step?' Thank you, Kathy, for your positivity and belief in me. The next step to me then actually creating this book came from working with one of the most patient, smart, kind and pragmatic women I've had the joy to meet – the incredible Kelly Irving. Kelly, your never-ending belief in me, your patience with my endless questions, edits and changes, your time, energy and wisdom, and your challenging questions and ideas are what made this book what it is. Thank you for helping me turn my dream into a reality. You are quite simply amazing. To Alex at Murdoch, I knew the moment I met you that you 'got it' and knew exactly what I wanted this book to be about and who it was for. You championed this book from the moment the manuscript landed on your desk, and I thank you from the bottom of my heart for that. To Sam and Virginia, for your endless editing advice I thank you so much. You have helped so much to shape my ideas and thoughts into a structure that lands so well – thank you.

This is a book about hope, and about going against the norm of societal conditioning to create a different life. I can't write acknowledgements without mentioning the people who helped me to get sober. Some of you I have never met in real life and yet have had such a profound impact on me, especially in the early days. To Mandy Manners and Kate Baily, authors of *Love Sober* and hosts of the podcast of the same name – the community you created in those early days got me sober. Thank you. To my Sober Spring sisters from the spring of 2018 – Kate, Kate, Nicole, Sophie and Simone. I wouldn't be sober without you. To Clare Pooley for your amazing book *The Sober Diaries* and for being such a support to me since I launched my coaching business.

Friendships change and evolve especially as we transition through different stages of life. If we find friends who can move through everything with us, still hold our hand and offer us support, even if it's not *their* journey, they are keepers for life. Love them hard. I am so lucky to have four of them: Coley, Chris, Paula and Kath. Where would I be without our 'Birthday Love' WhatsApp group?! From the clubs of Clapham in 1998 (yes, Infernos, I'm looking at you!) through to the present day, we have laughed, cried, championed, cheered and supported each other through it all. Maintaining closeness and love in friendships when we all live on opposite sides of the world takes effort, commitment and dedication and I am so proud of us all for the never-ending supply of love and support we show each other. One day the five of us will all be together soon and won't that be a day to celebrate! Special thanks go to Carla and Suzanne – thank you for taking pity on the weird Scottish girl with the bad perm back in 1989. To my girls here on the ground in Perth for the laughter, love, adventure and joy you bring to my life each and every week. You know who you are; thank you for everything.

When I launched my coaching business in early 2021, I could never have believed it would go on to support so many women. While so many people say to me, 'Sarah, I don't know how you do it all', the fact is, I don't. I have the most incredible team who have helped me build a business that supports thousands. Special thanks to Carmen, Eli, Amy, Evie and Ellie for your ongoing love, support and never-ending commitment to my mission in our business.

To my family – my mum, dad, Paul and Alice. Thank you for always having my back. Dad, you always encouraged me to think big and dream big. You instilled in me a belief I could do and be anything I wanted. You planted the seed for my passion to travel and it was because of you that I left home at 24 with a bag on my back to see the world. Mum, your kind heart, patient ear and endless cups of tea with biscuits have seen me through the toughest of times. You've watched me push every boundary and limit out there and always provided a soft place to land when it didn't go how I wanted. Those teenage years weren't easy but somehow we made it! Paul and Alice – the safety and security you have always offered me through even the most troublesome times has saved me more than you will ever know. Walking into your warm, loving home feels like coming home to me – it's the only place I ever want to be when the shit hits the fan. I just wish you were round the corner. Thank you for never judging and always offering a kind and supportive ear when I need it most.

To my husband Gus. From those backpacking days in Kalbarri, I can't quite believe the path we have travelled and where we are today. Your patience, your support and your belief in me are what push me each and every day to be the best version of myself. You never hold me back, you never laugh at my crazy ideas, you simply let me be and join me for the ride. I couldn't ask for anything more in a life partner. Thank you. I love you.

To Scarlett and Will. Everything I do, I do it for you. Thank you for being my greatest teachers. I wouldn't be sober if it wasn't for you. Reach for the stars, my darling children, the world is yours for the taking.

And, finally, to my ladies. You know who you are. Thank you for trusting me to be your guide and your coach. Thanks for your honesty and openness, and the love and commitment you show not just yourselves but each other. Our community is one of my proudest achievements in life and it's because of you. So many of you say to me, 'Sarah you changed my life,' and I always say, 'No, *you* changed your life, I just showed you the way.' But now I want to say to each and every one of you that you really have changed *my* life. Supporting and championing you fills my heart with joy each and every day. Thank you. I see you. I honour you. I am you.

ENDNOTES

My story so far ...

1. Page xiv '*I ordered the book and made a pledge to myself.*' Grace, A., *This Naked Mind: Control alcohol*, London: HQ, 2017.

2. Page xv '*Is it any wonder that middle-aged women are drinking more than ever?*' Roberts, L., 'Katie drinks more than she should. Research shows more middle-aged women are doing the same', ABC online, 27 January 2022, abc.net.au/news/2022-01-27/australian-risk-drinking-middle-aged-women-research-help/100783522

3. Page xv '*We are continually being sold the idea that alcohol is our "reward" at the end of a busy day ...*' Murray, J., 'The feminisation of alcohol marketing', BBC World Service, bbc.com/worklife/article/20200924-the-feminisation-of-alcohol-marketing

Chapter 1

1. Page 2 '*It was in the 1990s that the major alcohol companies began segregating their markets ...*' English, T., 'Why alcohol marketing targeting women has public health researchers concerned', WHYY, 24 April 2014, whyy.org/segments/why-alcohol-marketing-targeting-women-has-public-health-researchers-concerned

2. Page 3 '*... "Creating a successful marketing campaign for an alcohol brand is now a matter of activating experience at every touch point."*' The Sense Group, 2019, sensegroup.com.au/insights/experiential-marketing-for-alcohol-brands

3. Page 4 '*In a 2019 research article conducted by the Public Health Advocacy Institute of Western Australia, Curtin University, titled ...*' Public Health Advocacy Institute of Western Australia, Curtin University and Cancer Council WA, 'The "Instagrammability" of Pink Drinks: How alcohol is marketed to women in Australia', November 2019, eucam.info/wp-content/uploads/2019/11/PHAIWA-CCWA-The-Instagrammability-of-pink-drinks-How-alcohol-is-marketed-to-women-in-Australia-2019.pdf

4. Page 4 '*And it's working because more women are drinking at binge-drinking levels than ever before.*' Miller, M., Mojica-Perez, Y., Livingston, M., et al., 'The who and what of women's drinking: Examining risky drinking and associated socio-demographic factors among women aged 40–65 years in Australia', *Drug and Alcohol Review*, 26 January 2022, vol. 41 no. 4, pp. 724–31, doi.org/10.1111/dar.13428

5. Page 4 '*The report concluded that no amount of alcohol is safe and having any more than two drinks a week is risky.*' Paradis, C., Butt, P., Shield, K., et al., *Canada's Guidance on Alcohol and Health: Final report*, Ottawa, Ontario: Canadian Centre on Substance Use and Addiction, 2023, ccsa.ca/canadas-guidance-alcohol-and-health-final-report

6. Page 6 '*In fact, in a 2023 World Health Organization report titled "No level of alcohol consumption is safe for our health", it says ...*' Anderson, B.O., Berdzuli N., Ilbawi, A., et al., 'Health and cancer risks associated with low levels of alcohol consumption', *The Lancet Public Health*, January 2023, vol. 8 no. 1, e6–e7, doi.org/10.1016/S2468-2667(22)00317-6

7. Page 7 '*In fact, in the US alone, alcohol advertising spending in 2023 was set to hit US$7.7 billion.*' 'Big Alcohol Exposed: Big Investments in Advertising Onslaught', Movendi International, 28 May 2021, movendi.ngo/news/2021/05/28/big-alcohol-exposed-big-investments-in-advertising-onslaught

8. Page 7 '*In Australia, the most recent study (which was still twenty years ago) shows this spend to be in excess of $220 million ...*' White, V., Faulkner, A., Coomber, K., et al., 'How has alcohol advertising in traditional and online media in Australia changed? Trends in advertising expenditure 1997–2011', *Drug and Alcohol Review*, 19 June 2015, vol. 34 no. 5, pp. 521–30, doi.org/10.1111/dar.12286

9. Page 7 '*... and in the UK, if everyone drank the recommended units of alcohol each week ...*' Bhattacharya, A., Angus, C., Pryce, R., et al., 'How dependent is the alcohol industry on heavy drinking in England?', *Addiction*, December 2018, vol. 113 no. 12, pp. 2225–32, doi.org/10.1111/add.14386

10. Page 7 '*The specific marketing directed at young women in the UK from the early 90s coincided with an increase in the diagnosis of ...*' English, T., 'Why alcohol marketing trageting women has public health researchers concerned', WHYY, 24 April 2014, whyy.org/segments/why-alcohol-marketing-targeting-women-has-public-health-researchers-concerned

11. Page 8 '*David Jernigan, director of the Centre on Alcohol Marketing and Youth ...*' English, T., 'Why alcohol marketing trageting women has public health researchers concerned', WHYY, 24 April 2014, whyy.org/segments/why-alcohol-marketing-targeting-women-has-public-health-researchers-concerned

12. Page 8 '*And unsurprisingly for middle-aged women, binge-drinking and alcohol use disorder are only increasing.*' Miller, M., Mojica-Perez, Y., Livingston, M., et al., 'The who and what of women's drinking: Examining risky drinking and associated socio-demographic factors among women aged 40–65 years in Australia', *Drug and Alcohol Review*, May 2022, vol. 41 no. 4, pp. 724–31, doi.org/10.1111/dar.13428

13. Page 8 '*In terms of amounts of alcohol consumed, it is generally classed as ...*' 'Understanding Alcohol Use Disorder', National Institute on Alcohol Abuse and Alcohol, April 2023, niaaa.nih.gov/publications/brochures-and-fact-sheets/understanding-alcohol-use-disorder

14. Page 8 '*The Australian Bureau of Statistics classes binge-drinking as four or more standard drinks on one occasion ...*' 'Binge drinking (alcohol intoxication disorder)', Virtual medical centre, 23 April 2008, tinyurl.com/5n8rrmuw

15. Page 9 '*Gabor Maté, one of the world's leading specialists in addiction, as well as parenting ...*' Maté, G., 'How our childhood shapes every aspect of our lives', 'Motherkind' podcast, episode 65, June 2019.

16. Page 9 '*In fact, as revealed on the BBC Radio* Woman's Hour *show ...*' Murray, J., 'The feminisation of alcohol marketing', BBC World Service, bbc.com/worklife/article/20200924-the-feminisation-of-alcohol-marketing

17. Page 9 '*A 2017 US study found that "alcohol use disorder among females skyrocketed ..."*' Grant, B.F., Chou, S.P., Saha, T.D., et al., 'Prevalence of 12-Month Alcohol Use, High-Risk Drinking, and *DSM-IV* Alcohol Use Disorder in the United States, 2001-2002 to 2012-2013: Results From the National Epidemiologic Survey on Alcohol and Related Conditions', *JAMA Psychiatry*, 9 August 2017, vol. 74 no. 9, pp. 911–23, doi.org/10.1001/jamapsychiatry.2017.2161

18. Page 9 *'And in Australia, a study in the 2022* Drug and Alcohol Review *showed one in five Australian women ...'* Roberts, L., 'Katie drinks more than she should. Research shows more middle-aged women are doing the same', ABC online, 27 January 2022, abc.net.au/news/2022-01-27/australian-risk-drinking-middle-aged-women-research-help/100783522

19. Page 10 *'Women are more deficient in the key metabolising enzyme alcohol dehydrogenase (ADH) ...'* Franzen, H., 'Enzyme Lack Lowers Women's Alcohol Tolerance', Scientific American, 16 April 2001, scientificamerican.com/article/enzyme-lack-lowers-womens

20. Page 10 *'This explains why cognitive deficits, heart issues and liver disease occur earlier in women than men with significantly shorter exposure to alcohol.'* The Alcohol Pharmacology Education Partnership, 'Gender Differences in Alcohol Metabolism', Duke University Medical Center, North Carolina School of Science & Mathematics, sites.duke.edu/apep/module-1-gender-matters/content/content-gender-differences-in-alcohol-metabolism

21. Page 10 *'As alcohol dissolves in water, alcohol is more concentrated in a female body than a male body.'* Harvard Health Publishing, 'Ask the doctor: Why does alcohol affect women differently?', 1 January 2013, health.harvard.edu/womens-health/why-does-alcohol-affect-women-differently

22. Page 10 *'Depending on the time of the month and how high our oestrogen is at any given point ...'* University of Illinois at Chicago, 'Higher estrogen levels linked to increased alcohol sensitivity in brain's "reward center"', ScienceDaily, 7 November 2017, sciencedaily.com/releases/2017/11/171107092906.htm

23. Page 10 *'The Alcohol and Drug Foundation of Australia reported a study that one in ten breast cancer diagnoses in Australia ...'* Pandeya, N., Wilson, L., Webb, P., et al., 'Cancers in Australia in 2010 attributable to the consumption of alcohol', October 2015, vol. 39 no. 5, pp. 408–13, doi.org/10.1111/1753-6405.12456, as cited in 'Alcohol and Breast Cancer', Alcohol and Drug Foundation, 16 October 2022, tinyurl.com/mu8bba42

24. Page 10 *'Further afield, the World Health Organization stated in 2021 ...'* 'Alcohol is one of the biggest risk factors for breast cancer', World Health Organization, 20 October 2021, who.int/europe/news/item/20-10-2021-alcohol-is-one-of-the-biggest-risk-factors-for-breast-cancer

25. Page 12 *'When I interviewed Kathryn Elliott, a breast cancer survivor ...'* Written interview conducted by author, 22 June 2023.

26. Page 12 *'The Cancer Council of Australia also states that alcohol is related to ...'* 'Alcohol and cancer', Cancer Council NSW, cancercouncil.com.au/cancer-prevention/alcohol/alcohol-and-cancer

27. Page 12 *'Dr Helena Popovic, a leading authority on improving brain function ...'* Popovic, H., *Can Adventure Prevent Dementia?: A guide to outwitting Alzheimer's*, Canberra: Choose Health, 2023.

28. Page 12 *'To put this into context, COVID-19 was responsible for 6000 a day ...'* Written interview conducted by author 30 August 2022.

29. Page 14 *'Addiction expert Gabor Maté describes it as ...'* Maté, G., 'The Power of Addiction and the Addiction to Power', Mad in America, 23 March 2022, madinamerica.com/2022/03/the-power-of-addiction-and-the-addiction-to-power-gabor-mate-md

30. Page 15 *'This view was prevalent even back in the 1930s …'* 'More About Alcoholism' in *Alcoholics Anonymous: Big book*, New York, NY: Alcoholics Anonymous World Services, first published in 1939, p. 33, aa.org/sites/default/files/2021-11/en_bigbook_chapt3.pdf

31. Page 15 *'… Dr Nick Sheron, a liver specialist in the UK who said only one in three …'* Gray, C., *Sunshine Warm Sober: The unexpected joy of being sober forever*, London: Octopus, 2021.

32. Page 16 *'According to a study carried out by David Nutt, Director of the Neuropsychopharmacology Unit …'* Nutt, D., King, L.A., Saulsbury, W., et al., 'Development of a rational scale to assess the harm of drugs of potential misuse', *The Lancet*, 24 March 2007, vol. 369 no. 9566, pp. 1047–53, doi.org/10.1016/S0140-6736(07)60464-4

33. Page 16 *'Grey area drinking is a term coined by Jolene Park …'* Park, J., 'Gray Area Drinking', 2017, youtube.com/watch?v=wvCMZBA7RiA&t=2s

34. Page 19 *'Clare Pooley's book,* The Sober Diaries, *has a brilliant analogy of the early part of sobriety …'* Pooley, C., *The Sober Diaries: How one woman stopped drinking and started living*, London: Coronet, 2017.

Chapter 2

1. Page 27 *'In the sober world, we talk about the three Ms of alcohol use …'* Vargus, E., 'Heart of the Matter' podcast, season 3, episode 6.

2. Page 29 *'It says: "If you bring forth what is within you, what you bring forth will save you. If you do not bring forth what is within you, it will destroy you."'* Gospel of Thomas, verse 70, discovered in 1945, first published in English in 1956.

3. Page 30 *'In his book* Recovery: Freedom from our addictions, *author Russell Brand describes sugar …'* Brand, R., *Recovery: Freedom from our addictions*, Macmillian US, 2017.

4. Page 31 *'As Dr Pamela Stewart, a psychiatrist at the Centre for Addiction and Mental Health in Canada …'* as cited in Johnston, A.D., *Drink: The intimate relationship between women and alcohol*, New York, NY: Harper Wave, 2014, p. 108

5. Page 35 *'William Porter, in his book* Alcohol Explained, *describes this well when he writes: "Fading affect bias essentially describes …"'* Porter, W., *Alcohol Explained: Understand why you drink and how to stop*, Scotts Valley, CA: CreateSpace Independent Publishing Platform, 2015.

6. Page 36 *'Professor of Psychology Dr Judith Grisel says: "There is no good evidence that shows you can go back to moderate use after being addicted."'* As cited in Gray, C., *Sunshine Warm Sober: The unexpected joy of being sober forever*, London: Octopus, 2021.

7. Page 36 *'And Professor David Nutt, who specialises in addiction …'* As cited in Gray, C., *Sunshine Warm Sober: The unexpected joy of being sober forever*, London: Octopus, 2021.

8. Page 37 *'… "If I enjoy my drinking, I can't control it and if I control my drinking, I don't enjoy it."'* Jones, D., 'Florence Welch says "sobriety is the best thing I ever did"', NME Australia, 21 July 2022, nme.com/en_au/news/music/florence-welch-says-sobriety-is-the-best-thing-i-ever-did-3274325

9. Page 40 *'As Paul Dillon, the director and founder of Drug and Alcohol Research and Training Australia …'* Dillon, P., 'Doing Drugs With Paul Dillon' podcast, episode 5, 10 March 2022.

10. Page 40 *'We never learn to "sit in the shit" as my gorgeous friend …'* Buttress, A., 'Behind the smile with Ash Butterss', interview conducted with author.

11. Page 41 '*In Ann Dowsett Johnston's brilliant book,* Drink, *she says that daughters of alcoholic mothers are much more likely to develop problematic drinking habits themselves ...*' Johnston, A.D., *Drink: The intimate relationship between women and alcohol*, New York, NY: Harper Wave, 2014, p. 197.

12. Page 43 '*However, I have learnt through extensive reading and from my own experience of therapy that while these events describe "Big T" trauma ...*' Barbash, E., 'Different Types of Trauma: Small "t" versus large "T"', Psychology Today, 13 March 2017, psychologytoday.com/au/blog/trauma-and-hope/201703/different-types-trauma-small-t-versus-large-t

13. Page 44 '*In the now famous 1995 Adverse Childhood Experience (ACE) study ...*' Hammers-Crowell, J., 'Understanding the Connection Between Addiction and Trauma', Safe Harbor Recovery Center, 13 May 2019, safeharborrecovery.com/understanding-connection-addiction-trauma

14. Page 44 '*From the study we now know that an individual who experiences ...*' Nagata, J., Smith, N., Sajjad, O.M., et al., 'Adverse childhood experiences and sipping alcohol in U.S. children: Findings from the Adolescent Brain Cognitive Development Study', *Preventive Medicine Reports*, vol. 32 no. 102153, April 2023, doi.org/10.1016/j.pmedr.2023.102153

15. Page 44 '*He said, "The first question is not why the addiction but why the pain?"*' Malcom, L., Willis, O., 'Changing the way we think about addiction', ABC Radio, 27 August 2015.

Chapter 3

1. Page 51 '*While it takes 72 hours for alcohol to physically leave ...*' Sheppard, S., 'Dopamine and Addiction Recovery: Here's What You Should Know About the "Pleasure Chemical"', The Temper, 2 May 2019, thetemper.com/dopamine-addction-recovery

2. Page 52 '*Normally in the second half of our monthly cycle, when progesterone is at its highest ...*' Gilfarb R.A., Leuner, B., 'GABA System Modifications During Periods of Hormonal Flux Across the Female Lifespan', *Frontiers in Behavioral Neuroscience*, 16 June 2022, vol. 16 no. 802530, doi.org/10.3389/fnbeh.2022.802530

3. Page 52 '*As we age, however, our progesterone naturally starts declining from our late 30s onwards ...*' Roche, D., 'What Causes Low Progesterone Levels in Women?' Lets Get Checked, 17 February 2020, letsgetchecked.com/articles/what-causes-low-progesterone

4. Page 52 '*Initially alcohol mimics the effects of GABA ...*' Davies, M., 'The role of GABAA receptors in mediating the effects of alcohol in the central nervous system', *Journal of Psychiatry and Neuroscience*, 1 July 2003, vol. 28 no. 4, pp. 263–74, jpn.ca/content/28/4/263.short

5. Page 52 '*A study on the impact of alcohol on our neurotransmitters reveals that ethanol ...*' Banerjee, N., 'Neurotransmitters in alcoholism: A review of neurobiological and genetic studies', *Indian Journal of Human Genetics*, January–March 2014, vol. 20 no. 1, pp. 20–31, doi.org/10.4103/0971-6866.132750

6. Page 52 '*In order to reclaim that balance ...*' Porter, W., *Alcohol Explained: Understand why you drink and how to stop*, Scotts Valley, CA: CreateSpace Independent Publishing Platform, 14 April 2015, p. 41.

7. Page 53 '*As William Porter says in his book ...*' Porter, W., *Alcohol Explained: Understand why you drink and how to stop*, Scotts Valley, CA: CreateSpace Independent Publishing Platform, 14 April 2015.

8. Page 53 *'Ironically, one of the issues with long-term and consistent alcohol use is that our GABA receptors …'* Liang, J., Suryanarayanan, A., Abriam, A., et al., 'Mechanisms of Reversible GABAA Receptor Plasticity after Ethanol Intoxication', *The Journal of Neuroscience*, 7 November 2007, vol. 27 no. 45, pp. 12367–77, doi.org/10.1523/JNEUROSCI.2786-07.2007

9. Page 53 *'As Andrew Huberman, Associate Professor of Neurobiology at Stanford School of Medicine, explains …'* Huberman, A., 'What alcohol does to your body, brain and health', 'Huberman Lab' podcast, episode 22, August 2022, podcastnotes.org/huberman-lab/episode-86-what-alcohol-does-to-your-body-brain-health-huberman-lab

10. Page 54 *'The toxic effects of alcohol initially increase serotonin so we can experience …'* Lovinger D., 'Serotonin's role in alcohol's effects on the brain', *Alcohol Health Research World*, 1997, vol. 21 no. 2, pp. 114–20, pubmed.ncbi.nlm.nih.gov/15704346

11. Page 54 *'And just like GABA, while initially producing feelings of happiness and wellbeing, the long-term use of alcohol …'* Liang, J., Suryanarayanan, A., Abriam, A., et al., 'Mechanisms of Reversible GABAA Receptor Plasticity after Ethanol Intoxication', *Journal of Neuroscience*, 7 November 2007, vol. 27 no. 45, pp. 12367–77, doi.org/10.1523/JNEUROSCI.2786-07.2007

12. Page 54 *'Something else to consider when it comes to serotonin is that …'* Barandouzi, Z.A., Lee, J., del Carmen Rosas, M., et al., 'Associations of neurotransmitters and the gut microbiome with emotional distress in mixed type of irritable bowel syndrome', *Science Report*, 31 January 2022, vol. 12, no. 1648, doi.org/10.1038/s41598-022-05756-0

13. Page 54 *'It's actually a major cause of leaky gut and plays a key role in killing our good bacteria …'* Myers, A., 'Alcohol and Gut Health: Is Drinking Disrupting Your Microbiome?', amymyersmd.com/article/alcohol-gut-health

14. Page 55 *'Andrew Huberman says you can look around a room of teenagers …'* Huberman, A., 'What alcohol does to your body, brain and health', 'Huberman Lab' podcast, episode 22, August, 2022.

15. Page 55 *'Alcohol works in much the same way as other chemicals and behaviours that …'* Lewis, R., Florio, E., Punzo, D., et al., 'The Brain's Reward System in Health and Disease', *Advances in Experimental Medicine and Biology*, 13 November 2021 vol. 1344, pp. 57–69, doi.org/10.1007/978-3-030-81147-1_4

16. Page 57 *'The steps below are inspired by Deb Dana's book …'* Dana, D., Porges, S., *Polyvagal exercises for safety and connection: 50 client-centred practices*, New York, NY: W.W. Norton & Company, 2020.

17. Page 58 *'Andrew Huberman describes addiction as …'* Huberman, A., 'How Addiction Destroys Your Motivation', The Huberman Notes, Medium, 25 October 2022, medium.com/@henrik.moe.eriksen/how-addiction-destroys-your-motivation-28fbed2ff512

18. Page 60 *'REM is the cycle associated with dreaming and an incredibly important part of brain health …'* Jee, H.J, Shin, W., Jung, H.J., et al., 'Impact of Sleep Disorder as a Risk Factor for Dementia in Men and Women', *Biomolecules and Therapeutics (Seoul)*, 1 January 2020, vol. 28 no. 1, pp. 58–73, doi.org/10.4062/biomolther.2019.192

19. Page 60 *'Yet, scientists have found that when we drink, even just a little …'* 'Alcohol and sleep', *Drinkaware*, 1 November 2022, tiny.cc/f2v9vz

20. Page 60 *'Lack of REM sleep is linked to obesity, poor learning, low mood, poor heart health and dementia.'* Pase, M.P., Himali, J.J., Grima, N.A., et al., 'Sleep architecture and the

risk of incident dementia in the community', *Neurology*, 19 September 2017, vol. 89 no. 12, pp. 1244–50, doi.org/10.1212/WNL.0000000000004373

21. Page 60 '*When we are sedated, we switch off brain cells that would ordinarily be firing during the deep sleep stage ...*' Colrain, I.M., Nicholas, C.L., Baker, F.C., 'Chapter 24 - Alcohol and the sleeping brain', *Handbook of Clinical Neurology*, 2014, vol. 125, pp. 415–31, doi.org/10.1016/B978-0-444-62619-6.00024-0

22. Page 60 '*Neuroscientist and sleep specialist Matthew Walker has a brilliant talk ...*' Walker, M., 'How caffeine and alcohol affect sleep', Sleeping with Science, 2020, youtube.com/watch?v=KQ9FfzMKBNc

23. Page 60 '*Fragmented sleep can lead to increased fat mass, increased inflammation, increased insulin resistance ...*' Poroyko, V., Carreras, A., Khalyfa, A., et al., 'Chronic Sleep Disruption Alters Gut Microbiota, Induces Systemic and Adipose Tissue Inflammation and Insulin Resistance in Mice' *Scientific Reports*, 14 October 2016, vol. 6 no. 35405, doi.org/10.1038/srep35405

24. Page 60 '*Alcohol is also known to increase our hot flushes if we are in perimenopause ...*' Serrel, N., 'Does Alcohol Cause Hot Flashes?', The Guardian Recovery Network, 15 December 2022, tinyurl.com/ans7kjx3

25. Page 61 '*These dilated blood vessels can lead to the skin ...*' Freedman, R.R., 'Menopausal hot flashes: Mechanisms, endocrinology, treatment', *The Journal of Steroid Biochemistry and Molecular Biology*, July 2014, vol. 142, pp. 115–20, doi.org/10.1016/j.jsbmb.2013.08.010

26. Page 61 '*For women experiencing hot flushes as a result of hormone fluctuation in menopause ...*' Serrel, N., 'Does Alcohol Cause Hot Flashes?', Guardian Recovery Network, 15 December 2022, tinyurl.com/ans7kjx3

27. Page 62 '*When we add alcohol to the mix, it means our liver has to work overtime.*' 'Love Your Liver', Liver Foundation, liver.org.au/your-liver/about-the-liver/2022

28. Page 62 '*What's more concerning is that an increase in circulating oestrogen ...*' Travis, R.C., Key, T.J., 'Oestrogen exposure and breast cancer risk', *Breast Cancer Research*, 1 October 2003, vol. 5 no. 239, pp. 239–47, doi.org/10.1186/bcr628

29. Page 62 '*One study shows that drinking alcohol increases circulating oestrogen in the blood by over 20 per cent.*' Al-Sader, H., Abdul-Jabar, H., Allawi, Z,. et al., 'Alcohol and Breast Cancer: The Mechanisms Explained', *Journal of Clinical Medicine Research*, August 2009, vol. 1 no. 3, pp. 125–31, doi.org/10.4021/jocmr2009.07.1246

30. Page 62 '*According to Avonne Connor, Assistant Professor of Epidemiology at Johns Hopkins University ...*' Connor, A., 'Alcohol and Breast Cancer Risk', 'Breast Cancer Risk' podcast, 5 November 2021, breastcancer.org/podcast/alcohol-and-risk

31 Page 62 '*It's also really important to mention that when a woman hits the perimenopause years ...*' Brady, C.W., 'Liver disease in menopause', *World Journal of Gastroenterology*, 7 July 2015, vol. 21 no. 25, pp. 7613–20, doi.org/10.3748/wjg.v21.i25.7613

32. Page 62 '*There is so much we still don't know about the menopause years and the effect it's having on our body ...*' Brady, C.W. 'Liver disease in menopause', *World Journal of Gastroenterology*, 7 July 2015, vol. 21 no. 25, pp. 7613–20, doi.org/10.3748/wjg.v21.i25.7613

33. Page 63 '*In fact, women going through menopause are twice as likely to develop liver disease as men.*' McCarthy, C., 'Women with Menopause at Significantly Higher Risk of Developing NAFLD', Endrocrineweb, 25 January 2023, pro.endocrineweb.com/

endocrinology-news/with-menopause-women-at-significantly-higher-risk-of-developing-nafld

34. Page 65 *'Sleeping with a phone by our bed makes our brain more hypervigilant ...'* Gurarie, M., '3 Reasons To Avoid Using Your Phone In Bed', Health, 27 August 2023, health.com/mind-body/3-reasons-not-to-sleep-with-your-phone-in-your-bed

35. Page 67 *'The World Health Organization advises we have no more than twelve teaspoons in a day ...'* 'Sugar', Food Standards Australia New Zealand, August 2019, foodstandards.gov.au/consumer/nutrition/Pages/Sugar.aspx

36. Page 68 *'Schooner or pint of beer/ale = up to 9 teaspoons of sugar ...'* 'Calories and alcohol', Drinkaware, drinkaware.ie/facts/calories-and-alcohol

37. Page 69 *'Add in lots of dark green veggies ...'* Gunnars, K., 'How Much Water Should You Drink Per Day?', Healthline, 5 June 2023, healthline.com/nutrition/how-much-water-should-you-drink-per-day#how-much-you-need

38. Page 69 *'Feeding our good gut bacteria and starving our bad gut bacteria ...'* Spector, T., *The Diet Myth: The real science behind what we eat*, London: Orion, 2020.

39. Page 69 *'(Vitamin D supports our neurotransmitter production, particularly serotonin.)'* Anjum, I., Jaffery, S.S., Fayyaz, M., et al., 'The Role of Vitamin D in Brain Health: A Mini Literature Review', Cureus, 10 July 2018, vol. 10 no. 7, e2960, doi.org/10.7759/cureus.2960

40. Page 70 *'Dr Helena Popovic says that drinking three alcoholic drinks a night depletes our levels ...'* Popovic, H., *Can Adventure Prevent Dementia? A guide to outwitting Alzheimer's*, Canberra: Choose Health, 2023, p336.

41. Page 71 *'In fact, exercise has been shown to treat ...'* Pedersen, B.K., Saltin, B., 'Exercise as medicine – evidence for prescribing exercise as therapy in 26 different chronic diseases', *Scandinavian Journal of Medicine & Science in Sports*, December 2015, vol 25 no. 3, pp. 1–72, doi.org/10.1111/sms.12581

42. Page 72 *'A Boston University School of Medicine study found that ...'* 'How Meditation Boosts Anti-Anxiety Neurotransmitters: Serotonin & GABA', EOC Institute, tinyurl.com/5n97yb56

Chapter 4

1. Page 78 *'The World Health Organization calls it the greatest health risk of the 21st century ...'* Fink, G., 'Stress: The Health Epidemic of the 21st Century', Elsevier SciTech Connect, 26 April 2016, tinyurl.com/3shx75ap

2. Page 78 *'More and more research is revealing the impact stress plays in diseases ...'* 'Stress Symptoms: Effects on your body and behaviour', Mayo Clinic, 10 August 2023, tinyurl.com/29ta6as3

3. Page 78 *'When I interviewed Dr Wendy Sweet (PhD) ...'* Sweet, W., email conversation with author on 10 June 2023.

4. Page 83 *'As we saw earlier, this stress response state is called ...'* Nunez, K., 'Fight, Flight, Freeze: What This Response Means', Healthline, 10 February 2023, healthline.com/health/mental-health/fight-flight-freeze

5. Page 84 *'When we end up staying stuck in the sympathetic state for too long ...'* Todd, W., *SD Protocol: Achieve greater health by learning to balance your physical, chemical and emotional wellbeing*, ebook, 2016.

6. Page 91 '*In his book* The Body Keeps the Score ...' van der Kolk, B., *The Body Keeps the Score: Mind, brain and body in the healing of trauma*, London: Penguin, 2014.

7. Page 93 '*This term, coined by Dan Siegel, author and Clinical Professor of Psychiatry at the UCLA School of Medicine* ...' Siegel, D., *The Developing Mind: How relationships and the brain interact to shape who we are*, New York, NY: Guildford Publications, 1999.

8. Page 98 '*As a qualified practitioner, Sharon describes breathwork as* ...' Jennings, S., sharonjennings.com.au

9. Page 101 '*Jay Fields is an educator, coach and author who has taught the principles of embodied social and emotional intelligence* ...' Fields, J., jay-fields.com/about-jay-fields

10. Page 102 '*We know that one 60-minute meditation increases our GABA levels* ...' Streeter, C.C., Jensen, J.E., Perlmutter, R.M., et al., 'Yoga Asana Sessions Increase Brain GABA Levels: a Pilot Study', *The Journal of Alternative Complementary Medicine*, 28 May 2007, vol. 13 no. 4, pp. 419–26, doi.org/10.1089/acm.2007.6338

11. Page 102 '... *people who meditate regularly sleep better.*' Rusch, H.L., Rosario, M., Levison, L.M., et al., 'The effect of mindfulness meditation on sleep quality: a systematic review and meta-analysis of randomized controlled trials', *Annals of the New York Academy of Sciences*, June 2019, vol. 1445 no. 1, pp. 5–16, doi.org/10.1111/nyas.13996

Corliss, J., 'Mindful meditation helps fight insomnia, improves sleep', Harvard Health blog, 15 June 2015, health.harvard.edu/blog/mindfulness-meditation-helps-fight-insomnia-improves-sleep-201502187726

12. Page 102 '*A podcast hosted by Dr Rangan Chatterjee, author and influential British GP, offered the following advice* ...' 'Feel Better, Live More with Dr Rangan Chatterjee', BBC radio, episode 23.

13. Page 104 '*There is much evidence now to suggest the positive impact of cold water therapy on reducing stress.*' Espeland, D., de Weerd, L., Mercer, J.B., 'Health effects of voluntary exposure to cold water – a continuing subject of debate', *International Journal of Circumpolar Health*, December 2022, vol. 81 no. 1, e2111789, doi.org/10.1080/2242 3982.2022.2111789

Huttunen, P., Kokko, L., Ylijukuri, V., 'Winter swimming improves general well-being', *International Journal of Circumpolar Health*, May 2004, vol. 63 no. 2, pp. 140–4, doi.org/10.3402/ijch.v63i2.17700

14. Page 104 '*You only have to look at the popularity of practitioners like Wim Hof.*' Kopplin, C.S., Rosenthal, L. 'The positive effects of combined breathing techniques and cold exposure on perceived stress: a randomised trial', *Current Psychology*, 7 October 2022, vol. 42, pp. 27058–70, doi.org/10.1007/s12144-022-03739-y

15. Page 104 '*In fact, Dr Andrew Huberman says that starting your day with cold* ...' Huberman, A., 'The Science & Use of Cold Exposure for Health & Performance' Huberman Lab, 1 May 2022, hubermanlab.com/the-science-and-use-of-cold-exposure-for-health-and-performance

Huberman, A., 'Controlling Your Dopamine for Motivation, Focus & Satisfaction', 'Huberman Lab' podcast, episode 39.

16. Page 104 '*There is also evidence to suggest that doing hot yoga (yoga in a deliberately hot studio) significantly reduces symptoms of depression.*' Nyer, M., Hopkins, L.B., Farabaugh, A., et al., 'Community-Delivered Heated Hatha Yoga as a Treatment for Depressive

Symptoms: An Uncontrolled Pilot Study', *The Journal of Alternative and Complementary Medicine*, 15 August 2019, vol. 25 no. 8, pp. 814–23, doi.org/10.1089/acm.2018.0365

17. Page 107 '... *I highly recommend* Accessing the Healing Power of the Vagus Nerve ...' Rosenberg, S., *Accessing the Healing Power of the Vagus Nerve: Self-help exercises for anxiety, depression, trauma, and autism*, Berkeley, CA: North Atlantic Books, 2017.

Chapter 5

1. Page 113 '*Dr Libby Weaver, one of Australasia's leading nutritional biochemists, encapsulates this perfectly in her book ...*' Weaver, L., *Rushing Woman's Syndrome: The impact of a never-ending to-do list and how to stay healthy in today's busy world*, London: Hay House, 2017.

2. Page 114 '*In my coaching, I ask my clients to complete Gretchen Rubin's 'The Four Tendencies Quiz ...*' Rubin, G., 'The Four Tendencies Quiz', gretchenrubin.com/quiz/the-four-tendencies-quiz

3. Page 114 '*Gabor Maté covers this in detail in his book ...*' Maté, G., *The Myth of Normal: Trauma, illness & healing in a toxic culture*, London: Random House, 2022.

4. Page 114 '*He also states that 80 per cent of all people diagnosed with autoimmune conditions are women.*' Maté, G., 'The Untold Truth Why 80% of Autoimmune Sufferers are Women', 2023, youtube.com/watch?v=taYVjQ0_ldA

5. Page 115 '... *something Maté says cannot be linked to genetics or diet and instead attributes to the increased stress ...*' 'Trauma, Illness and Healing with Gabor Maté', 'Feel Better, Live More' podcast with Dr Rangan Chatterjee, BBC radio September, 2022.

6. Page 115 '*Because the woman was absorbing the stress of her partner.*' Weiyao, Y., Ludvigsson, J.F., Åden, U., et al., 'Paternal and maternal psychiatric history and risk of preterm and early term birth: A nationwide study using Swedish registers', *Plos Medicine*, 20 July 2023, vol. 20 no. 7, e1004256, doi.org/10.1371/journal.pmed.1004256

7. Page 115 '*Contemporary studies have shown that women took on more emotional stress during the pandemic ...*' Ding, Y., Yang, J., Ji, T., et al., 'Women Suffered More Emotional and Life Distress than Men during the COVID-19 Pandemic: The Role of Pathogen Disgust Sensitivity', *International Journal of Environmental Research and Public Health*, 12 August 2021, vol. 18 no. 16, e8539, doi.org/10.3390/ijerph18168539

8. Page 115 '*It's no wonder we also saw a correlation with a rise in women's drinking ...*' White, A., Castle, I-J.P., Chen, C.M., et al., 'Converging Patterns of Alcohol Use and Related Outcomes Among Females and Males in the United States, 2002 to 2012', *Alcoholism Clinical and Experimental Research*, 1 September 2015, vol. 39 no. 9, pp. 1712–26, doi.org/10.1111/acer.12815

9. Page 116 '*And there is also this from Bessel van der Kolk in his book* The Body Keeps the Score ...' van der Kolk, B. *The Body Keeps the Score: Mind, brain and body in the transformation of trauma*, London: Penguin, 2014.

10. Page 118 '*In her book* The Top Five Regrets of the Dying, *palliative nurse Bronnie Ware shares the top five regrets ...*' Ware, B., *The Top Five Regrets of the Dying: A life transformed by the dearly departing*, Carlsbad, CA: Hay House, 2019.

11. Page 131 '*James Clear's book* Atomic Habits *is the bible for creating new habits ...*' Clear, J., *Atomic Habits: An easy & proven way to build good habits & break bad ones*, New York, NY: Random House, 2018.

Chapter 6

1. Page 148 '*I conducted a poll in one of the alcohol-free challenges I ran ...*' In January 2023 I ran an alcohol-free challenge with over 650 women from all over the world.

2. Page 148 '*Studies show that some women under the influence of alcohol ...*' Cooper, M.L., O'Hara, R.E., Martins J., 'Does Drinking Improve the Quality of Sexual Experience?: Sex-Specific Alcohol Expectancies and Subjective Experience on Drinking Versus Sober Sexual Occasions', *AIDS and Behaviour*, 16 July 2015, vol. 20 no. 1, pp. 40–51, doi.org/10.1007/s10461-015-1136-5

3. Page 148 '*According to research in the National Library of Medicine, alcohol use causes testosterone to drop.*' Emanuele, M.A., Emanuele, N.V., 'Alcohol's Effects on Male Reproduction', *Alcohol Health and Research World*, 1998, vol. 22 no. 3, pp. 195–201, ncbi.nlm.nih.gov/pmc/articles/PMC6761906

   Koh, K., Kim, S.S., Kim, J.S., et al., 'Relationship between Alcohol Consumption and Testosterone Deficiency according to Facial Flushes among Middle-Aged and Older Korean Men', *Korean Journal of Family Medicine*, 20 November 2022, vol. 43 no. 6, pp. 381–7, doi.org/10.4082/kjfm.21.0173

4. Page 149 '*As Jacqueline says, "Mature sex takes its time, appreciates all aspects of the experience ..."*' Hellyer, J., '#348: Sex Should Age Like A Fine Wine', 12 February 2023, jacquelinehellyer.com/lovelife_blog/sex-should-age-like-a-fine-wine

5. Page 154 '*In his book* The Seven Principles for Making Marriage Work, *author and Professor of Psychology John Gottman says ...*' Gottman, J., Silver, N., *The Seven Principles for Making Marriage Work: A practical guide from the country's foremost relationship expert*, New York, NY: Harmony, 2015.

6. Page 157 '*However, according to the team at Resurgence Behavioral Health, "over 70 per cent of people on top dating apps drink ..."*' '8 Best Sober Dating Apps for People in Recovery', Resurgence Behavioral Health, 26 August 2022, resurgencebehavioralhealth.com/blog/8-best-sober-apps-for-people-in-recovery

Chapter 7

1. Page 165 '*Something that helped me so much with this complex and often highly emotional stage in my sobriety was the passage ...*' Passaro, J., *A Good Man: Every man will make a mistake, few will have an impact*, Scotts Valley, CA: CreateSpace Independent Publishing Platform, 2015.

2. Page 166 '*You may also have heard the famous quote ...*' Chalker, B., 'A reason, a season, a lifetime', oncommonground.wordpress.com/2008/10/09/a-reason-a-season-a-lifetime

3. Page 169 '*In his book* Necessary Endings, *Dr Henry Cloud writes ...*' Cloud, H., *Necessary Endings: The employees, businesses, and relationships that all of us have to give up in order to move forward*, New York, NY: HarperCollins, 2010.

4. Page 170 '*More and more places are starting to stock alcohol-free drinks ...*' Allen, M., 'Why more alcohol-free drinks are now pouring at a venue near you', Financial Review, 17 June 2022, tinyurl.com/3p3jurr6

5. Page 172 '*Dr Swart describes our connections to these five people as crucial and states that ...*' Swart, T., *The Source: Open your mind, change your life*, London: Random House, 2020.

6. Page 177 *'Johann Hari says in his famous TEDx talk …'* Hari, J., 'Everything you think you know about addiction is wrong', 2015, ted.com/talks/johann_hari_everything_you_think_you_know_about_addiction_is_wrong?language=en

7. Page 177 *'Hari also describes loneliness and lack of human connection …'* Sapozhnikov, I., 'Lost Connections: Uncovering the Real Causes of Depression – and the Unexpected Solutions' *The Permanete Journal*, 1 September 2019, vol. 23 no. 3, p. 18–231, doi.org/10.7812/TPP/18-231

Chapter 8

1. Page 182 *'As author Mark Manson puts it …'* Manson, M., 'Why I Quit Drinking Alcohol', markmanson.net/why-i-quit-drinking-alcohol

2. Page 183 *'Dr Anna Lembke, the author of* Dopamine Nation, *says …'* Lembke, A., *Dopamine Nation: Finding balance in the age of indulgence*, London: Headline, 2023.

3. Page 186 *Of course, I didn't recognise this was happening, but psychologists tell us that …'* Lipton, B., 'How we are programmed at birth', 2018, tinyurl.com/bdd5bnwc

4. Page 191 *'As Helen Keller said: "Life is either a daring adventure or nothing at all."'* Keller, H., *The Open Door*, New York, NY: Doubleday, 1957.

5. Page 194 *'With that in mind, I want to introduce …'* Fredrickson, B., *Positivity: Top-notch research reveals the 3-to-1 ratio that will change your life*, New York, NY: Harmony, 2009.

6. Page 194 *'This quote by author and Associate Professor at Hardin-Simmons University Melissa Madeson …'* Madeson, M., 'Seligman's PERMA+ Model Explained: A Theory of Wellbeing', Positive Psychology, 24 February 2017, positivepsychology.com/perma-model

7. Page 196 *'In his book* Deep Work, *author and Professor of Computer Science Cal Newport talks about the fact that the human brain actually …'* Newport, C., *Deep Work: Rules for focused success in a distracted world*, New York, NY: Grand Central Publishing, 2016, pp. 212–13.

8. Page 197 *'Our subconscious brain is more susceptible to new thoughts in the first twenty minutes after waking …'* Schneider, J., 'A Neuroscientist's Morning Routine Doesn't Begin Without This Brain-Healthy Habit', 9 August 2023, mindbodygreen.com; tinyurl.com/4hus9yzy

9. Page 198 *'There is a brilliant podcast episode featuring anxiety expert Dr Jodi Richardson and Dr Helena Popovic …'* Richardson, J., 'Well hello anxiety with Dr Jodi Richardson', podcast, episode 88, 7 June 2023.

10. Page 200 *'Being in nature and taking in the shapes created in snowflakes, clouds, streams, coastlines, lakes and raindrops …'* Lambrou, P., 'Fun with fractals? Why nature can be calming', *Psychology Today*, 7 September 2012, tinyurl.com/yc8crpcs

11. Page 203 *'The advertising strategy of major companies to ensure we buy their products is to induce FUD …'* Tharakan, K.M., 'How to Ethically Market with FUD: Fear, Uncertainty, & Doubt', Strategy Peak, strategypeak.com/fud-fear-uncertainty-doubt

Chapter 9

1. Page 214 '*As author and founder of the Be Sober online community Simon Chapple says in his book* …' Chapple, S., *How to Heal Your Inner Child: Overcome past trauma and childhood emotional neglect*, London: Sheldon Press, 2021.
2. Page 219 '*If you're interested in creating your own morning routine* …' Elrod, H., *The Miracle Morning: The 6 habits that will transform your life before 8am*, London: John Murray, 2016.

RESOURCES

For more information and additional resources, visit my website sarahrusbatch.com/beyond-booze-resources

Chapter 2
Podcasts
Feel Better, Live More with Dr Rangan Chatterjee and Gabor Maté, 'How Our Childhood Shapes Every Aspect of Our Health', episode 37.

Rich Roll with Gabor Maté, 'How Trauma Fuels Disease', episode 702.

Unlocking Us with Brené Brown and Dr Marc Brackett, 'Permission to Feel', April 2020.

Therapy
National Register of Schema Therapists, 'Schema Therapy', stia.com.au/national-register

Books
The Body Keeps the Score: Mind, brain and body in the transformation of trauma, Bessel van der Kolk, Penguin UK, 2014.

Happy Days: The guided path from trauma to profound freedom and inner peace, Gabrielle Bernstein, Hay House US, 2022.

In the Realm of Hungry Ghosts: Close encounters with addiction, Gabor Maté, Random House UK, 2018.

The Myth of Normal: Trauma, illness & healing in a toxic culture, Gabor Maté, Random House UK, 2022.

Permission to Feel: Unlock the power of emotions to help yourself and your children thrive, Dr Marc Brackett, Quercus UK, 2019.

When the Body Says No: The cost of hidden stress, Gabor Maté, Scribe Publications AU, 2019.

Websites
News in Health, 'Dealing With Trauma', June 2018, newsinhealth.nih.gov/2018/06/dealing-trauma

Chapter 3
Podcasts
Huberman Lab with Andrew Huberman, 'Leverage Dopamine to Overcome Procrastination & Optimize Effort', episode 39.

Huberman Lab with Andrew Huberman, 'What Alcohol Does to Your Body, Brain & Health', episode 86.

Books
Alcohol Explained: Understand why you drink and how to stop, William Porter, CreateSpace Independent Publishing Platform US, 2015.

Boundless: Upgrade your brain, optimize your body & defy aging, Ben Greenfield, Victory Belt Publishing US, 2020.

Dopamine Nation: Finding balance in the age of indulgence, Dr Anne Lembke, Headline UK, 2023.

Glucose Revolution: The life-changing power of balancing your blood sugar, Jessie Inchauspé, Simon & Schuster US, 2022.

Websites

BravermanTest.net, 'Neurotransmitters', bravermantest.net

Dr Helena Popovic, drhelenapopovic.com

MyMT by Dr Wendy Sweet (PhD), 'My Menopause Transformation', 2023, mymenopausetransformation.com

Chapter 4

Therapy

'About Dr. Peter Levine', Somatic Experiencing Australia, seaustralia.com.au/what-is-somatic-experiencing/dr-peter-levine

Australian Breathwork Association, australianbreathworkassociation.org.au

International Breathwork Federation, ibfbreathwork.org

'Shaking (Live Your Life with Devotion)', Qoya, youtube.com/watch?v=-yUzux2lR_Q

'Tension and Trauma Releasing Exercises (TRE™)', TRE Star Groups, youtube.com/watch?v=2qx63W496Uo&feature=emb_logo

Books

Accessing the Healing Power of the Vagus Nerve: Self-help exercises for anxiety, depression, trauma, and autism, Stanley Rosenburg, North Atlantic Books US, 2017.

SD Protocol: Achieve greater health and wellbeing, Wayne Todd, BookBaby, 2016.

Waking the Tiger: Healing trauma, Peter Levine, North Atlantic Books US, 1997.

Websites

Jay Fields, jay-fields.com

Liz McComish, embodime.com.au

Sharon Jennings, sharonjennings.com.au

Apps

Insight Timer, insighttimer.com

Chapter 5

Podcasts

'Feel Better, Live More' with Dr Rangan Chatterjee and Gabor Maté, 'Trauma, Illness and Healing in a Toxic Culture', episode 294.

Books

Atomic Habits: An easy & proven way to build good habits & break bad ones, James Clear, Random House US, 2018.

The Myth of Normal: Trauma, illness & healing in a toxic culture, Gabor Maté, Random House UK, 2022.

Set Boundaries, Find Peace: A guide to reclaiming yourself, Nedra Glover Tawwab, Piatkus UK, 2021.

Setting Boundaries: Care for yourself and stop being controlled by others, Dr Rebecca Ray, Pan Macmillan AU, 2021.

Chapter 6
Books
The Seven Principles for Making Marriage Work: A practical guide from the country's foremost relationship expert, John Gottman, Nan Silver, Harmony US, 2015.
Websites
The Gottman Institute, 'The Gottman Method', gottman.com/about/the-gottman-method
Jacqueline Hellyer, jacquelinehellyer.com
Apps
Clean and Sober Love, cleanandsoberlove.com
Loosid, loosidapp.com
Meet Mindful, meetmindful.com
Meetville, meetville.com
Single and Sober, singleandsober.com

Chapter 7
Books
Fair Play: A game-changing solution for when you have too much to do (and more life to live), Eve Rodsky, Hachette AU, 2019.
Find Your Unicorn Space: Reclaim your creative life in a too-busy world, Eve Rodsky, Hachette AU, 2021.
Websites
To find out what alcohol-free drinks are available, check out sarahrusbatch.com/alcohol-free-drinks
Social sober groups
Club Soda, @joinclubsoda, joinclubsoda.com/about-club-soda
Perth Sober Socials (Facebook group), facebook.com/groups/1093211501076062
Soberistas, soberistas.com
Untoxicated, untoxicated.com.au
The Women's Wellbeing Collective, thewomenswellbeingcollective.org

Chapter 8
Inspirational people I follow
Andrew Huberman, hubermanlab.com
Craig Harper, craigharper.net
Davina McCall, thisisdavina.com
Davinia Taylor, instagram.com/daviniataylor/?hl=en
Gabby Bernstein, gabbybernstein.com
Glennon Doyle, momastery.com
Dr Helena Popovic, drhelenapopovic.com
The Holistic Psychologist, theholisticpsychologist.com
James Clear, jamesclear.com
Dr Julie Smith, doctorjuliesmith.com
Libby Weaver, drlibby.com
Mel Robbins, melrobbins.com
Dr Mindy Pelz, drmindypelz.com
Pippa Campbell, pippacampbellhealth.com

Dr Rangan Chatterjee, drchatterjee.com
Dr Wendy Sweet, mymenopausetransformation.com
Dr Will Cole, drwillcole.com
Zoe Blaskey, motherkind.co

Chapter 9
Podcasts
'Behind the Smile', Ash Butterss
'Feel Better Live More', Dr Rangan Chatterjee
'Huberman Lab', Andrew Huberman
'The Mel Robbins Podcast', Mel Robbins
'Motherkind', Zoe Blaskey
'Sober Awkward', Vic and Hamish
'This Naked Mind', Annie Grace
'Well Hello Anxiety', Dr Jodi Richardson
'The You Project', Craig Harper

Books
Conscious Loving: The journey to co-committment, Gay Hendricks, Kathlyn Hendricks, Random House US, 1992.

Drink: The intimate relationship between women and alcohol, Ann Dowsett Johnston, HarperCollins AU, 2013.

Happy Mind, Happy Life: 10 simple ways to feel great every day, Dr Rangan Chatterjee, Penguin UK, 2022.

Lost Connections: Why you're depressed and how to find hope, Johann Hari, Bloomsbury UK, 2019.

The Power of Now: A guide to spiritual enlightenment, Eckhart Tolle, Hachette AU, 2011.

Quit Like A Woman: The radical choice to not drink in a culture obsessed with alcohol, Holly Glenn Whitaker, Bloomsbury UK, 2020.

The Sober Diaries: How one woman stopped drinking and started living, Clare Pooley, Coronet UK, 2017.

Stolen Focus: Why you can't pay attention, Johann Hari, Bloomsbury UK, 2023.

The Unexpected Joy of Being Sober, Catherine Gray, Octopus UK, 2017.

We Are the Luckiest: The surprising magic of a sober life, Laura McKowen, New World Library US, 2020.

ABOUT THE AUTHOR

Since removing alcohol from her own life in April 2019, Sarah has dedicated her life to supporting women like her, stuck in the grey area drinking cycle, to break free and reclaim their lives, as well as spreading her two core messages: 'a life without alcohol is not boring' and 'you don't have to be an "alcoholic" to decide to quit booze'.

Sarah is an accredited grey area drinking coach, health and wellbeing coach, menopause coach and a passionate advocate for women's health and happiness, especially in midlife. She works with women across the globe through her alcohol-free programs and her self-discovery group coaching programs which allow women to discover 'who the hell they really are' without alcohol. Sarah also speaks on stages across Australia and, more recently, in the corporate world on the topic of 'grey area drinking', a new term so few people are familiar with.

Sarah has featured in multiple television, radio and podcast interviews, as well as print interviews such as *Mamamia*, *The Sydney Morning Herald*, the *Daily Mail*, *Red Magazine*, *Body and Soul* and Channel 9 news, sharing her own journey to sobriety as a message of hope to other women who feel stuck, and also her opinions on 'Mummy wine culture' and the impact alcohol messaging is having on women's health.

Originally from Manchester in the UK, Sarah has lived in Perth, Western Australia, since 2010 with her husband, two children, mad cocker spaniel, and ruler of the house – Striker the cat.

Sarah speaks from the heart and will never stop on her mission to support, empower and champion women all over the world and of all ages to live lives that are fulfilling, rich, diverse and interesting without the need for the numbing effects of alcohol.

CONNECT WITH ME

I'm a girl's girl through and through and love nothing more than connecting with like-minded women across the globe. Don't be shy!

You can email me: hello@sarahrusbatch.com

Visit my website for all the ways I work with women all over the world: sarahrusbatch.com

Join my incredible community of women at The Women's Wellbeing Collective: facebook.com/groups/342319476897067

Follow me on Instagram at instagram.com/sarahrusbatch

Follow me on Facebook at facebook.com/sarahrusbatchcoach

I am on a mission to help as many women as possible create a life they love, alcohol-free. If you would like to support me in this goal, you can do so by reviewing this book on any of the major book websites such as Amazon, Booktopia and Goodreads. This helps us reach more women. Together we are stronger! Thank you so much.

INDEX

oestrogen 61, 62, 85
oestrogen dominance 62
operating systems, to support values 217–23, 227
others, meeting the needs of 113–17, 120
oxytocin 185

parasympathetic nervous system 82, 105, 106
parasympathetic state 84, 86, 88–9, 94, 95
parents, behaviour of 39–41, 92, 125
Park, Joelene 16
partners *see* relationships
Passaro, John A. 165–6
past traumas 21
people trees 172–3
perimenopause 60–1, 62, 79
phenylalanine 73
pink drinks 4
pistachios 65
podcasts 45
polyvagal theory 101
Pooley, Clare 19
Popovic, Helena 12, 70, 198
pornography 55
Porter, William 35, 53
positive emotions 194–202, 206
positives, looking for 56–8
Positivity (Fredrickson) 194
pregnancy 5, 115
premenstrual tension 31–2
pride 195–6, 233
procrastination 87
progesterone 51–2
Prosen, Lisa Villa 200
Public Health Advocacy of Western Australia 4
purpose, in life 224–6

questioners 114
quitting *see* sobriety

rapid eye movement (REM) sleep 60
Raye (singer) 29
reading 72

rebels 114
Recovery: Freedom from our addictions (Brand) 30
reflection 118–19
reflexology 106
reiki 106
relationships
  boundaries in 126–7
  checking in with partners 144–6
  for single women 157–8
  navigating changes in 140–1, 159
  openness and honesty in 140–3
  rituals shared with partners 150–2, 154, 221
  separation from a partner 156–7
  sex 148–50, 160, 161
  shared interests and goals 154–6
  sobriety and relationships 137–61
  understanding and communicating needs 146–8
  see also friends; parents
REM sleep 60
responsibility 232–4
'responsible drinking' 16
rest and digest branch, nervous system 82, 84, 89
Resurgence Behavioural Health 157
rheumatoid arthritis 114–15
Richardson, Jodi 198
rituals, shared with partners 150–2, 154, 221
role modelling 38–41, 43, 117–18, 140
Rosenberg, Stanley 107
Rottnest Island 167
Rubin, Gretchen 114
running 180
Rushing Women's Syndrome (Weaver) 113

sadness, drinking to avoid 31
saunas 104
screen time 127, 220–1
sedative effect, of alcohol 60
self, boundaries for 127
self-care 112, 127, 205, 219, 221–2
self-compassion 202
self-growth 221